Medical Imaging Methods

Medical Imaging Methods

Theory and Applications

Edited by
Ashutosh Kumar Shukla

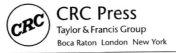

CRC Press
Taylor & Francis Group
Boca Raton London New York

CRC Press is an imprint of the
Taylor & Francis Group, an **informa** business

First edition published 2022
by CRC Press
6000 Broken Sound Parkway NW, Suite 300, Boca Raton, FL 33487-2742

and by CRC Press
2 Park Square, Milton Park, Abingdon, Oxon, OX14 4RN

© 2022 Taylor & Francis Group, LLC

CRC Press is an imprint of Taylor & Francis Group, LLC

ISBN: 9780367630812 (hbk)
ISBN: 9780367630799 (pbk)
ISBN: 9781003112068 (ebk)

DOI:10.1201/9781003112068

Typeset in Minion
by Deanta Global Publishing Services, Chennai, India

Dedicated to COVID-19 frontline health workers

Contents

Preface

Medical imaging is a field of societal interest including professionals. This collection has six chapters covering different aspects of medical diagnosis and imaging. These chapters are spread over a wide range from the benefits and risks of X-ray imaging to artificial intelligence applications in different imaging techniques. A particular chapter is included to review cone beam tomography applications in dentistry. Two chapters present the nanoparticle applications in medical imaging and the role of nanobiosensors. Computer-aided diagnosis and artificial intelligence applications dealing with ethical issues are covered in two chapters. These chapters not only present the review but also connect the reader to new clinical indications.

I am thankful to the reviewers for their wonderful suggestions, especially to the reviewer who suggested that the ethical issue should appear on top. I realized the importance of this suggestion while going through the chapters and have incorporated this suggestion with satisfaction. My sincere thanks are due to the expert contributors from different countries who have woven the content in a manner suitable for the interdisciplinary audience. They contributed in a timely manner and helped me a lot to meet the schedule.

I would like to thank Shivangi Pramanik, Commissioning Editor – Medicine, CRC Press, and Himani Dwivedi, Editorial Assistant – Medical, CRC Press, for their constant support during different stages of publication.

Ashutosh Kumar Shukla
Ewing Christian College, Prayagraj

About the Editor

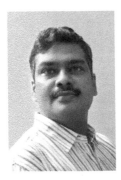

Dr Ashutosh Kumar Shukla is an Associate Professor of Physics at Ewing Christian College, Prayagraj, a constituent college of University of Allahabad, India. Being an enthusiastic academician, and with about 20 years of physics teaching and research experience, he has to his credit publications in peer-reviewed journals, review articles, textbooks, and several edited volumes prepared in areas such as medicine, food science, archaeology and cultural heritage, crude oil, and water quality analysis in collaboration with experts from different countries. Dr Shukla has successfully completed research projects and presented his research in different international events organized in different countries. He is on the reviewer panel for many international journals and is a member of the International EPR Society (IES) and web member of the International Society of Magnetic Resonance (ISMAR). Dr Shukla has received prestigious fellowships including the Bilateral Exchange Fellowship and the Visiting Fellowship of Indian National Science Academy, New Delhi.

Contributors

Zühre Akarslan
Oral and Maxillofacial Radiology
    Department
Faculty of Dentistry
Gazi University
Ankara, Turkey

Megha P. Arakeri
Center for Imaging Technologies
M. S. Ramaiah Institute of Technology
Bangalore, India

Nursel Arpay
Oral and Maxillofacial Radiology
    Department
Faculty of Dentistry
Gazi University
Ankara, Turkey

Octavian G. Duliu
Faculty of Physics
Department of Structure of Matter,
    Earth and Atmospheric Physics and
    Astrophysics
University of Bucharest
Bucharest, Romania

Lakshmana
Reva University
Bangalore, India

Chandra Rekha Makanjee
Discipline of Medical Radiation Sciences
Faculty of Health
University of Canberra
Canberra, Australia

Sunil Kumar Manvi
Reva University
Bangalore, India

Monalisa Mishra
Neural Developmental Biology Lab
Department of Life Science
NIT Rourkela
Rourkela, Odisha, India

Reetuparna Nanda
Neural Developmental Biology Lab
Department of Life Science
NIT Rourkela
Rourkela, Odisha, India

Pratyusha Nayak
Neural Developmental Biology Lab
Department of Life Science
NIT Rourkela
Rourkela, Odisha, India

Peter M. Ndangili
School of Chemistry and Material
    Science (SCMS)
Technical University of Kenya
Nairobi, Kenya

Naumih M. Noah
School of Pharmacy and Health Sciences
United States International
    University-Africa (USIU-A)
Nairobi, Kenya

Hatice Tetik
Oral and Maxillofacial Radiology
    Department
Faculty of Dentistry
Gazi University
Ankara, Turkey

Diagnostic Medical Imaging Services with Myriads of Ethical Dilemmas in a Contemporary Healthcare Context
Is Artificial Intelligence the Solution?

Chandra Rekha Makanjee

Introduction

Modern diagnostic medical imaging (DMI) is complex, with access to multiple digital imaging modalities and techniques available. DMI methods supported by digital general radiographic and fluoroscopy systems, high-sensitivity detectors with quantum detection, advanced algorithms eliminating motion artefacts, and medical imaging monitors with a resolution of three to eight megapixels significantly differ from conventional screen film radiographic methods. Then current innovative technological advancement in computed tomography (CT), magnetic resonance imaging (MRI), isotopic methods, ultrasonography using elastography, and new solutions in doppler imaging are focused on reducing radiation exposure with better imaging capabilities and throughput (1).

DOI: 10.1201/9781003112068-1

This evolution reflects the utilization of complex ionizing and non-ionizing DMI technologies simultaneously, resulting in a constant flux in the diagnostic medical imaging healthcare professionals' (DMIHCP) roles and responsibilities. This is mediated through technology including the social, biomedical, and psychological context, influenced by advances in the fields of physics, medicine, biology, and engineering and including innovations in computer and data sciences (2). This means working with a diverse range of medical and non-medical healthcare professionals (HCP) in achieving and ensuring equitable access to a timely diagnosis and quality outcomes for the person as the patient. In an artificial intelligence (AI) context, this can be achieved by using smart data analytics in patient scheduling, decision support for safe and appropriate order entry, natural language processing-based querying and annotation of radiology reports, resource utilization dashboards, and the prediction of healthcare economic trends. With neural networks capable of self-learning, constant and autonomous improvement and refinement of workflows can take place in the background. So, there is a shift in tasks that can yield larger net efficiencies, rather than mere pixel-based computer-aided detection tools (3).

From a healthcare systems perspective the DMIHCPs' functioning extends well beyond the recognition of pathological patterns in images. DMIHCPs routinely employ "real" intelligence to convert accurate image interpretation into actionable, holistic patient-centric decision-making in variable medical settings ranging from office-based outpatient private imaging centres to tertiary academic research hospitals with a complex case mix and comorbid patients whose care as already mentioned involves multidisciplinary team consultations and involvement in problem solving. Further DMI services are distributed across various level of healthcare systems consisting of engineers, non medical and medical healthcare providers, physicists, technological specialist hence inherently interdependent in nature to achieve a seamless quality health outcomes.

An integral component of the aforementioned is the ethical aspect. Professional ethics is the basis for each professional's work, as it includes values and principles, together with rights and duties that guide and support professionals (4). As stated earlier, DMI is inherently interdependent with a diverse range of HCPs both medical and non-medical to function effectively in achieving a timely diagnostic outcome, as well as seamless quality of patient care as the person as the patient journeys through the healthcare system. The ethics of each profession is important as collaboration and interdependencies increase (5) in an already complex evolving health system environment. DMI occupy an exceptional space and it serves an integral role in medicine. The rapid development and expansion of DMI have produced indisputable benefits to patients in terms of life expectancy and quality of life. Taking into consideration this inherent distributed diverse, and temporal nature of DMI services within a medical encounter and the ease of access, one cannot ignore the associated harm or risks with a referral for a diagnostic medical imaging examination (DMIE) and the outcomes thereof within the safety context. To practice medical imaging within a health system context at an exceptional level entails providing an effective and efficient culturally safe care and services.

The Distributed Nature of Medical Imaging Services

The best possible diagnostics, patient care, and care outcomes require multidisciplinary competences and thus interprofessional collaboration (4). Engineers, IT technicians, and physicists, among others, provide unique expertise to a DMI within a medical encounter (5).

Enabling a seamless DMI service requires effective communication, meticulous cooperation, coordination, and collaboration through each point of contact with the patient and the HCP and between HCPs from the point of referral to the outcomes of their clinical diagnosis in mapping their treatment and management plans for the patients as persons within a health system context. Simultaneously, the process must be aligned with the organization's goals, objectives, and values and professional regulatory body practice standards and professional code of conduct. So, each team member must have a collective understanding of the task at hand as their direct or indirect contribution is interdependent and interrelated with other team members as the patient journeys through and navigates various pathways of the healthcare system's processes and procedures to achieve a quality health outcome (see Figure 1.1).

It is relatively easy for a radiographer, nurse, doctor, physiotherapist, or other professional to work in isolation and do their job without giving much thought to the bigger picture like the rest of the hospital and the service that patients receive. The case is similar for the engineers, medical physicists, and maintenance teams who need to ensure that the equipment is optimal in its functioning and the physical structure is safe and hazard-free depending on the financial resources. So, to provide this seamless high-quality care requires members of a multidisciplinary team to stay focused on their specific tasks and contribution to bridge a potential gap in care or else inadequate health services may result, affecting the realization of the ethical principles of beneficence (6).

Demonstrating clear cause-and-effect relationships between collaborative team behaviour and particular outcomes is often difficult (7). Ideally, the team should work together successfully with equality and balance, no team member should seek to dominate the team, team members should have trust and confidence in one another's roles, responsibilities, and professional identity, and they should treat each other with respect, which Strudwick and Day call professional adulthood (5). Importantly, team members should recognize the

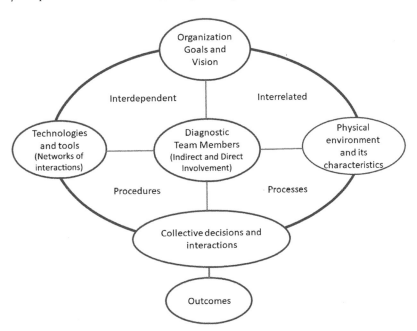

Figure 1.1 Illustrating the interconnectedness and interdependent nature of diagnostic medical imaging.

different value perspectives, moral commitments, and priorities of the differing professions on the team, and they should feel safe to share and to defer professional autonomy to another professional. Furthermore, problem solving should be open and honest, flexible adaptable and team members should be able to work across professional boundaries (4). Of importance is being familiar with and understand the appropriate profession or discipline specific with its used language and terminology. If any of the aforementioned is compromised, interprofessional jealousy and conflicts could arise. In reality tribalism is unavoidable because every profession has its own occupational culture which differs from others, resulting in in-group and out-group behaviour and a tendency to classify the profession as "us" (e.g., medical practitioners) and all other groups as "them" (e.g., allied health professionals such as nurses and radiographers and radiologists). "They" are "the other", and this "otherness" implies both differences and a different status. Most often the "other" (e.g., nurses and radiographers) is viewed as inferior or of less value than "us" (radiologists and medical practitioners) and is subject to stereotyping and prejudice (5).

As a typical example, the volume of radiology journal papers discussing, debating, and evaluating AI has increased exponentially since 2015 as radiologists quickly tackled initial concerns over role demise and extinction by writing counterarguments extolling the benefits of AI automation as an assistive and augmentative technology, not an existential threat. Radiographers are used to the fact that augmentation and support always focus on the radiologist rather than working together with the radiographers who are the mediators between the patient, referring medical practitioners (RMP), and the radiologist. One could argue that this upsurge in radiologist interest and debate was driven, in part, by role preservation and protectionism, but equally it has served as the voice that rationalized the value of the human worker within the imaging chain, a factor so easily overlooked in the quest for service and cost efficiencies (8). Frequently omitted both in clinical medicine and in radiology are the role and responsibilities of the radiographer often perceived as a mere button pusher.

This could be a lack of full awareness of the roles of other professionals, leading to prejudice and misunderstanding, and lastly mutual lack of education is often a cause of job tension. Newcomers to a profession construct a sense of their profession via legitimate peripheral participation and via discourse and learn their profession's duties, boundaries, values, and aspirations. It is often during moments of tension, and the exchanges that follow, that judgements about "others" are formed. To overcome the issue of interprofessional conflict, Wiles et al. suggest that rather than focusing on the tensions of the multidisciplinary team the focus should be on dilemmas in a patient's care. This means that rightness and wrongness are not necessarily determined by the actual outcome but by the quality of decisions and approaches used by the team in each situation because each team member involved might have different primary duties and concerns (6).

The Complex Medical Imaging Encounter and Associated Complexities

The DMIHCP's role as a clinician is complicated, involving much more than simply performing DMIE, DMI intervention procedures, applying imaging protocols and evaluating and interpreting images; it also includes the communication of findings where applicable, quality assurance, quality improvement, education, policy-making, and many other tasks that cannot be performed by computer programmes. The wisdom and experience of these DMIHCPs is difficult to quantify and even more difficult to simulate with AI systems. The question is whether that accountability can be relinquished. The ability to deal with DMIE not only entails the nuanced use of clinical judgement, but also functioning in a constant flux faced with technological changes and advancements which directly influence the profession and clinical practice in terms of rapidly adapting and adopting advanced imaging opportunities to operate new technologies. Further the value proposition of DMIHCPs extends to before a diagnostic image is taken, important information about patient safety, radiation protection, pre-test probability, appropriateness, study protocol, and patient preparation need to considered in terms of medical physics, epidemiology, and health system context. A key role of the DMIHCP with the patient prior to the DMIE is to check and verify identification and indications for the requested DMIE to explain and inform the patient about the procedure of the examination to be undertaken. During the actual DMIE the interaction is focused on acquiring cooperation from th patient and coordinate the examination in acquiring an optimal quality image series. Post-DIME entails interaction on the outcomes of the examination and, where contrast is administered, ensuring that the aftercare procedures are understood.

A quality decision is dependent on the field expert knowledge, competency, and confidence of the individual when faced with a particular situation. With regard to DMIE the decision taken at that point in time is based on an interaction with the patient and/or with another healthcare professional about the patient or in interactions with healthcare professionals or non-healthcare professionals (Table 1.1).

Irrespective, a golden thread here is the decision-making events, procedures and processes dependent on the relaying of information and messages with great efficiency and accuracy without losing their meaning; this is accomplished by the request order form, the efficiency with each the DMIE is conducted with optimal quality visual images that enable interpretation and evaluation to compile a report. Throughout these events one cannot ignore the ethical principles that govern daily practice. According to Mahmoodi and co-authors, collective decisions, e.g., jury verdicts, medical diagnosis, or financial investment, are often characterized by an uncertain choice between known alternatives (9). Information is exchanged, collectively explored, and adjusted at the patient's different points of contact in a medical encounter, and the outcomes of the various decision-making events are integrated and collectively reflected in the final diagnosis and treatment plan (10,11).

For example, at the point of initial assessment is the generation of an initial working diagnosis—usually a differential diagnosis—based on the initial clinical information. It may also include a referral for a screening DMIE. This is followed by the RMP/clinical team who decides whether DMIE is appropriate in the given clinical scenario, based on how likely imaging is to change the diagnosis in a meaningful way. Then one must take into consideration access and the availability of imaging modalities, additional data sources, such as additional history, observational data, and laboratory data where applicable. The determination of appropriateness is typically conducted primarily by the clinical team, though the decision often depends on input from the DMIHCP team with the use of an appropriate protocol based on the clinical scenario. Although the RMP/clinical team's request typically specifies the modality, the DMIHCP reviews the request, making recommendations for modifications as appropriate, and selects the specific imaging protocol to conduct the actual examination. Followed by the interpretation of the images with a radiology report that includes a summary of their findings and the likely implications for the given clinical scenario. Once the image is taken, then, the meaning of the image is interpreted with reference to the patient's condition and the referring doctor's needs. Analyzing and

Table 1.1 An Outline of the Interactions with the Diverse Team and the Patient of a DMI within a Medical Encounter

Activity	Question or Decision	Responsible Team	Patient Involvement
Initial assessment	What is the differential diagnosis according to the initial clinical information?	Clinical team	High: history, physical examination, discussion regarding working diagnosis
Imaging appropriateness determination	How is imaging likely to change the working diagnosis?	Clinical team with input from DIMHCP	Medium: discussion regarding appropriateness of imaging, patient-specific questions and concerns
Modality and protocol selection	Which imaging modality should be used? Specifically, how should it be performed?	DIMHCP with input from clinical team	Medium: image-specific questions, such as scheduling, contrast agent allergies, pregnancy status, patient identification, and so forth
Interpretation	What are the implications of the imaging findings, given the clinical scenario?	DIMHCP	Low: patient's perspective of clinical scenario, question to be answered
Integration	Based on the interpretation, what is the new working diagnosis?	Clinical team with input from DIMHCP	Medium: ongoing dialogue regarding revised working diagnosis
Goal alignment	What are the patient's realistic health outcome goals?	Patient and clinical team	High: understanding patient's perspective in the clinical context
Treatment determination	Based on the working diagnosis, what treatment would best achieve the desired outcomes?	Clinical team with input from and consent of patient	High: alignment of patient goals with treatment strategies, understanding of treatment goals, expectations for follow-up

interpreting an image entail integrating knowledge of false positives (arising from artefacts or false signals) and false negatives (anatomic pitfalls, heuristics, and cognitive biases that potentially lead to errors) with the timely communication of uncertainty, urgency, and unexpected findings (12). Throughout this process ethically sound judgement and decision-making processes are required in justifying the referral, conducting an optimal quality DMIE, and producing timely outcomes which add value to the quality health outcomes. In an evolving healthcare environment, all HCPs involved directly and indirectly must be fluent in the application of ethical concepts and ethical schools of thought and have an appreciation of the role of ethical practice in a clinical setting. Similarly, ethics also interacts with medical law to provide the safe and equitable delivery of healthcare (13).

Currently, the COVID-19 pandemic highlights the risks that can be involved in healthcare work. McDougal and others address the risks of healthcare work. The safety of HCPs is a pressing issue with clinical ethics questions faced by HCPs at the microlevel as they navigate patient care. Generally, in clinical ethics decision-making, choosing between different options involves balancing different values, obligations, or principles. The two critical values that need to be balanced are the duty to care for patients and personal well-being. These can sometimes be emotionally challenging, even frightening, ethical decisions to have to make, when one's own safety is involved and that of one's family. Whether conceived in terms of obligations to family members (12) or the intertwined interests of family members, keeping family members well is an important aspect of health professionals' personal well-being. There is no algorithm for calculating an ethically appropriate balance between optimal staff protection and optimal patient care. However, using a structured approach will enable situation-specific decision-making. It will also provide a basis for articulating the reasons for a decision, showing what assumptions and judgements were made. This sort of transparency and accountability is particularly important in ethically and emotionally challenging situations like those involving PPE in the COVID-19 pandemic (14).

Introducing AI in the DMI Context

Within healthcare, AI is an emerging constituent of many applications, including medical diagnostics and imaging. The value of AI is its speed and accuracy in the detection, segmentation, and classification of image features. Potential uses of narrow AI currently include tuberculosis and pneumonia detection in chest radiography, acute ischaemic stroke detection, and radiographic bone age assessment. Outside the confines of image interpretation, AI can potentially have an even larger positive effect on the non-interpretive but resource-intensive ancillary imaging processes that take place in the background—for example, scanner and hospital workflows, decision support, and retrospective studies (2). Unlike humans, it does not suffer from fatigue, forgetfulness, or the social limitations of prescribed working hours. The ethics behind the use of AI are complex; taking into consideration the rapid pace of AI development and issues of adaptation, adoption, and sustainability requires robust oversight and guidance that ensures ethical acceptance by its users and the recipients, namely the patients. It is important for DMIHCPs as well as other stakeholders to have the capability and ability to recognize the limitations and biases by identifying and applying AI's best features in an ethically appropriate way (15). This includes reviewing and parsing out the boundaries between the HCP and the machine's role in patient care and adjusting the education of future HCPs to proactively tackle the imminent changes within the profession's scope and practice. Also, opportunities for greater autonomy and self-definition require redefining clinical roles and responsibilities, educating IT-competent, multimodality professionals, and clinical workplace requiring competent skilled professionals. This implies that issues of role expansion such as cross-modality expertise and clinical flexibility need to be addressed.

Advanced virtual human avatars can engage in meaningful conversations, which has implications for the diagnosis and treatment of psychiatric disease. AI extends into the physical realm with robotic prostheses, physical task support systems, and mobile manipulators assisting in the delivery of telemedicine (11). In the DMI context Hardy and Harvey are of the opinion that direct human communication between patient and HCP is unlikely to be replaced by AI technologies (8). There is potential to enhance the automated vetting of DMI referrals and sense-checking clinical indications and the corresponding imaging modality and techniques to be employed, as well as verifying patient identification records via interaction with the electronic health record. It would require DMIHCPs to ensure patient electronic health record data are not corrupted and that AI decisions are consistent. Hence, all aspects pertaining to AI must be quality assured; AI-enabled systems must include quality control checks, regular audits, and reviews of the outputs and decisions of an AI image evaluation system. Also, it is necessary to factor in the many false negative and positive results needing correction.

The Basics of DMIE Ethical Principles

According to Malone and Zölzer, taking on board the contemporary thinking on social, medical, and ethical concerns, a set of principles/values should include respect for autonomy (of the individual), non-maleficence (do not harm), beneficence (do good), and justice is rooted in "common morality". Social expectations identify additional values which are also relevant for ethical decision-making in the DMIE context which are prudence (keeping in mind the possible long-term risks of actions) and honesty (sharing knowledge with those concerned truthfully) (16).

From a non-maleficence principle of medical ethics, ensuring patients' safety and preventing any injury or damage to them is a major priority for HCP. From a moral perspective, the main goal of patient safety can be studied as a practical value, where the emphasis is on the positive outcomes and benefits, and then as a moral value focusing on the protection and promotion of humanity and human dignity. From a professional point of view, moral values in patient safety are inseparable from basic medical obligations and a central source of other moral values emphasized in medicine. So patient safety is closely related to the concept of human dignity, and all patient safety measures taken must ensure the protection of human dignity. The responsibility of the HCS and professional commitment, in general, are closely related to human dignity (17). Hence the model for patient care, with caring as its central element, should integrate inherent ethical aspects (intertwined with professionalism) with clinical and technical expertise. It is not unusual that in patient care situations, there are conflicts between ethical principles (especially between beneficence and autonomy) (18).

In the medical context, the value of autonomy is to ensure that the patient is the main decision-maker in his or her own case. Consideration for the individual's point of view in some form is probably part of medical professional ethics globally. For example, within DMIE safety and protection context, wherever possible, the imposition of a risk must take account of the individual's volition as a prerequisite for justification (16). It is an integral part of the RMP's responsibility to adequately explain and inform the patient prior to the DMIE. Inadequate knowledge on DMIE makes it challenging for the RMP to inform patients about the risks and benefits of a DMIE. Without this information, the patient is unable to make an informed decision about alternative procedures based on the pros and cons of a particular procedure (19).

Then non-maleficence and beneficence are ethical principles, and it is important to be aware of the fact that they sometimes work against each other. It is best to treat others as you would like to be treated yourself could serve as a support for the principles of non-maleficence and beneficence. The value lies in considering everyone's interests as if they were your own (16).

The three related values are human dignity, prudence and honesty. Human dignity is more easily demonstrable as a cross-cultural concept than autonomy. As the world shrinks to a "global village", there is a need to develop approaches to decision-making that are acceptable for people from different cultural backgrounds. The principles proposed by Beauchamp and Childress can indeed be demonstrated in a wide range of cultural, religious and philosophical contexts. It appears in a contemporary form at the beginning of the United Nations Universal Declaration of Human Rights (16). DMI is, more than most medical activities, truly global in its clinical application, research base, industrial infrastructure, and regulatory framework. Patients and doctors travel and will find themselves in the presence of different cultural contexts. International organizations such as the World Health Organization, International Atomic Energy Agency, European Commission, and International Commission on Radiological Protection (ICRP) and numerous professional bodies must present their findings in language that is not alien to large groups of health professionals and lay populations throughout the world. So, everyone around the world could use as a form of moral guidance (16).

Where an action can potentially cause serious irreversible harm, measures to protect against it must be taken even if the causal relationships involved are not fully established scientifically. This is prudence or precaution. Lastly, honesty extends well beyond financial matters and includes openness and transparency about the benefits and risks of procedures. Justice, intergenerational equity, and inclusivity require that people are not deceived (see also section on AI) (16).

Value judgements on the appropriateness of a DMI procedure decision require knowledge of the implications of the act, and ethical and societal values. The three basic radiation protection and safety three pillars are the science of radiation protection, a set of ethical values, and experience accumulated from the daily practice of radiation protection by DMIHCPs. The three fundamental principles are justification, optimization, and individual dose limitation. The four ethical values are beneficence/non-maleficence, prudence, justice, and dignity. Quantifying benefits and harms is often problematic, and the threshold between an appropriate and an inappropriate act can vary among patients and patient groups. Ethics provide insights into the principles and philosophy of radiation protection and dialogue among all stakeholders to highlight values and preferences in view of a positive balance between potential benefits and harms.

Beauchamp and Childress developed four principles for biomedical ethics which forms building blocks for an ethics of radiological protection in medicine. They are: Respect for autonomy, the imposition of a risk has to take account of the individual's volition, and this is a prerequisite for justification. Non-maleficence and beneficence and justice as it asks everyone to consider the interests of the other as if they were his or her own. Within the DMI context, an examination which is unlikely to contribute to a positive health outcomes. May result in increase risk to unnecessary medical radiation exposure. Given the moral obligation of HCPs, the ethical indication is to lower the risk, ie, the benefit outweighing the risk, by considering the appropriateness of the prescribed DMIE and and optimally performed. At the same time, there is an ethical relevance related to the benefit to society, which is not achieved and quite disregarded if there is an unbalance between the health outcome and associated costs. Demand and supply are considered the main mechanisms at the base of over-imaging. The expanded availability of these examinations and increased demand from patients, together with demand from RMPs for assurance, could be perceived as a means to comfort patients and medical practitioners (MPs), where the benefits are easily overestimated, while risks and costs are somewhat neglected. Individual health assessment on radiation protection could also play a role in increasing unnecessary examinations. The attention to these ethical values may become a difficult task if the risks are uncertain, as for the low doses.

According to Salerno and others, decision-making under uncertainties requires prudence as a central value. Prudence should not be taken as synonymous with conservatism or "never taking risk", but it defines and sustains the way in which decisions are made, and it does not refer only to the outcome of those decisions. So, prudence represents the ability to make an informed and well-considered decision under uncertainty, without having full knowledge of the consequences of the undertaken action (20).

The justification principle combines the ethical values of beneficence and non-maleficence, with the ethical value of prudence. A prudent ethical practice accompanied by effective communication is part of justification, and it is important, where relevant, to avoid possible exposure to unnecessary radiation exposure. Justice, as a core value, requires equitable treatment for all. A proper DMIE, at the right time, with attention to justification and optimization, can have significant value for the patient and the society, whilst overutilization of DMIE leads to the inappropriate use of resources that could be used for other medical purposes, thus violating the justice in the distribution of services. Justice relates to our sense of fairness, like considering radiation risk by avoiding over-imaging paediatrics in view of their higher risk of adverse effects of radiation, compared with adults (20).

Honesty veracity, and truthfulness have therefore been suggested as guiding values for the interaction between specialists and lay people exposed to radiation. Accountability also arises as a matter of honesty that is relevant in the context of radiation protection (16).

Ethico-legal responsibility for decision-making remains in the hands (better, in the mind) of the natural intelligence of DMIHCPs. From this viewpoint, a multidisciplinary approach could take shared responsibility in difficult cases, considering the information AI provides as relevant but not always conclusive (21). Patients' preferences and values play a non-negligible role; human interaction and empathy from the DMIHCPs remain fundamental. Theoretically it is envisaged that AI will enable DMIHCPs to have more time to communicate with patients and to confer with colleagues in multidisciplinary teams, as they will be less busy doing routine and monotonous tasks that can be effectively performed by computers (22).

It is imperative that stakeholders develop a realistic sense of *how* AI is to be integrated in clinical practice and identify potential ethical pitfalls and possible solutions and offer policy recommendations on AI technology against the backdrop of striking a balance between the benefits and risks of AI technology as a complementary tool. For instance, from an interprofessional perspective, the focus has now shifted to the integration of complex machine learning algorithms and AI systems within equipment operation and image review processes.

It is difficult to balance and satisfy the values, beliefs, and opinions of diverse HCP involved in ethical choice. It is for the HCP to choose action or non-action, taking into consideration societal, civic, and professional values, including personal values. The rapid evolution of the healthcare environment impacts the ways in which moral/ethical problems are manifested. These changes may affect the manifest nature of the ethical and moral problems to be expected, but the domain of moral action is unaffected; the capacity to identify these new dilemmas relies on personal attributes such as one's moral values, sensitivity, and ethical vigilance.

Discussion, analysis, problem solving, and decision-making are critical to the ethical resolution of conflicts. It is important to define the problem, obtain a careful analysis of the facts (e.g., stakeholders involved or affected), check on the values involved in any possible decision or try to anticipate the implications of alternative decisions, evaluated costs and benefits of the ethical decision. Before undertaking an analysis, map out the situational context and the norms involved. Identify points of strength and place the ethical choice in its context. Of course, there is one's own experience, and the knowledge and skills acquired from professional training and continued education. Working in a professional network, with a participatory, multidisciplinary outlook to safeguard workers, and tackling the challenges posed by the contemporary work context.

Simultaneously consider every aspect that forms barriers to correct professional ethics such as conflicts of interest, failure to keep up to date, taking a "closed" attitude to one's own single discipline, and discrimination. On this last point, social morals may foster discrimination against certain categories of HCP, based on their sex, nationality, religion, or political beliefs.

The most important "next step" useful to resolve ethical challenges should include the development of a corpus of ethical principles that adequately consider the changing world of work, demographic shifts, new technologies, and, more generally, the impact of globalization. An ethics code must be current and relevant, providing indications for OHPs and serving as a reference point against which to measure one's own work. It must be incorporated in the curricula of both medical undergraduate and postgraduate ethics courses. Closely collaborate with OHPs and other key professionals. OHPs must seek the support and cooperation of employers, workers, and their organizations, including the competent authorities, professional and scientific associations, and other relevant national and international organizations, for implementing the highest standards of ethics in occupational health practice. Have scenarios highlighting ethical dilemmas which do not present easy policy choices. Scenarios are a useful instrument to provoke policy makers and other stakeholders, including industry, in considering the privacy, ethical, social, and other implications of the changing world of work, particularly new and emerging technologies (23).

An effective and precise correct application of AI may be powerful, helpful, and valuable only if considering the ethical implications such as the risks and harm associated with this cutting-edge technology for both patients and DMIHSPs. Factors to consider are security, privacy protection, and the ethical use of sensitive information to ensure both humane and regulated (and, therefore, responsible) management of the patients bound by core ethical principles, such as beneficence and respect for patients, which have guided clinicians during the history of medicine. To achieve a seamless use of AI requires all involved stakeholders to work collectively.

Multifaceted DMI Service Utilization Issues and Safety

The system of medical ionizing radiation protection and safety globally relies on the recommendations of the ICRP which is based on evidence-based value judgements that allow regulatory professional bodies and government institutions to develop policies and guidelines to seek solutions to practical problems in industry, medicine, education, research, and in everyday life and apply best practice principles. There are several research studies on assessing the awareness, concern, and practice on hazards of ionizing radiation and radiation protection among HCPs as well as patients. However, there is little recognition of radiation protection principles such as justification and optimization and dose limitation. On the other hand, many in healthcare environments misunderstand dose limitation obligations and incorrectly believe patients are protected by norms including a dose limit. These authors are also of the opinion that there is a deficiency in the educational training of HCPs (16).

The difficult justification process and issues utilization: the justification for a DMIE is not an easy task like writing a request order. The added value lies in quality services in patient care for timely diagnoses taking safety into consideration. Apart from the safety aspects, timely access, cost, and the competency and efficiency of the HCP involved directly and indirectly in deciding the most appropriate examination and the modality of choice must be considered. At the point of referral and when receiving the patient at the DMI section the shared responsibility of both the RMP and DMISP is to ensure that the requested DMIE is justified by outweighing the harm. The DMIE should be appropriate to answer the clinical question as well using a radiation dose that is as low as reasonably achievable (ALARA). This entails taking into consideration, for example, the radiation exposure time to which an individual is exposed.

Radiation sensitivity knowledge is essential when considering the justification process (24). RMPs should be knowledgeable about the biological effects of radiation as patients might present them with a history and signs of deterministic and stochastic effects. Always consider the use of non-ionizing radiation DMIE such as MRI or US. If the RMP is unaware of the doses and effective utilization of non-ionizing DMI modalities then the likelihood of inappropriate examinations is high, and an underestimation of radiation dose could result in an increased risk for both patients and DMIHCSPs (19, 24).

A lack of discrimination between ionizing and non-ionizing radiation examinations may lead to the poor justification of medical exposure. It also depends on the equity and equality of access to these services. A recent study demonstrates the DMIE ethical dilemma of paediatric patients with psychomotor development impairment when weighing the benefits versus the risks of that diagnostic or therapeutic procedure (25). For instance, children with cerebral palsy, who have a higher risk of low bone mass density, osteoporosis, and bone fractures, will be frequently referred for DMIE to monitor their hip migration to prevent dislocation, frequent injury, and bone/joint deformities. Exposing them to additional ionizing radiation such as DXA analysis poses an ethical dilemma because in comparison to the adult, paediatric exposure to ionizing radiation carries a greater risk of malignancy, especially leukaemia and thyroid cancer. These patients often undergo tests before or without consenting to a procedure and alternative diagnostic procedures are hardly discussed. The complexity arises because the effects of an exposure to these procedures could take 5 to 20 years to manifest.

It is imperative that one weigh moral and ethical judgement and commitment. The significant therapeutic opportunities in the field of prevention in this patient population from

DMIE outweigh the risks, where the ethical principle of beneficence becomes more binding than the principle of no maleficence (primum non nocere—do no harm). For example, the effective utilization of multiple exposures to DMIE reduces the risk of further damage to health, the onset of pain and suffering, a significant deterioration in the quality of life, and an additional shortening of the life expectancy of vulnerable paediatric patients such as those diagnosed with cerebral palsy.

In another example, central venous catheter (CVC) placement is a common procedure performed in the management of critically ill patients. CVC placement could result in associated risks such as malposition or iatrogenic pneumothorax. Though chest radiography has been the standard method to evaluate CVC position and to identify potential complications, diagnostic ultrasound has advantages because of the lack of ionizing radiation exposure, decreased resource utilization, and decreased diagnostic time. Timely clinical management could potentially affect patient outcomes (26). However, access to these services also depends on the cost involved and whether the sonographer is available, especially outside of normal working hours.

Issues of utilization: by definition, overutilization may be defined as the application of imaging procedures in clinical situations where imaging tests are unlikely to improve quality patient outcomes (27). Despite modest effects from initiatives such as the Choosing Wisely campaign, unnecessary DMIE remains a challenge (28). Key factors influencing imaging overuse include the practice behaviour of RMPs, self-referral (including referral for additional DMIE, duplicate imaging studies, defensive medicine, missed educational opportunities when inappropriate procedures are requested, patient demand, payment mechanisms, and financial incentives (as in the US healthcare system)) (24). Referrers' lack of knowledge of the roles and limitations, and unrealistic expectations of DI may lead to inappropriate imaging but also to false reassurance following a negative investigation. Besides the major financial and health consequences, includes further wasted efforts for unnecessary diagnosis and treatment and patient anxiety and individuals and the general population to unnecessary radiation doses. Much of the focus shifts to the management of incidentalomas rather than their adverse consequences which are difficult to capture in their entirety because unnecessary diagnostic hints could complicate the future care of a patient in unpredictable ways (29).

Defensive medicine: a widespread challenge in contemporary medicine relates to concerns about missing unexpected or rare findings, fear of litigation, avoiding an inaccurate diagnosis, or keeping costs low. There is also the question of confidence and competence among RMPs in diagnosis. RMPs with low confidence in clinical assessment over-rely on DMIE (30). Understanding the value of DMI should form an integral part of the framework of medical decision-making and the selection of the correct therapy. Unnecessary DMIE rarely reveals the cause of a patient's complaint, yet it may disclose incidental findings, which necessitate further imaging or interventional procedures to be clarified. DMI by itself does not improve patient health and provides no intrinsic value to patients. The risk includes false-positive and false-negative diagnoses and cannot be considered absolute. One must understand the information within the specific clinical context, for example the patient's history, previous DMIE, and other clinical data, to form an integrated whole that either confirms or excludes a given diagnosis. A confounding factor is the possible self-interest by stakeholders such as policy makers, payers, physicians, the imaging industry, and patients, resulting in ethical imperatives of trust and professionalism and conduct (27).

There is a tendency to rely on DMIE rather than clinically examining patients before requesting an examination found in the literature. The question is, will the patient judge the adequacy of or justification for DMIE referral? This practice could potentially expose patients to unnecessary radiation. Consulting the DMIHCP when uncertain of which DMIE to request prevents requesting inappropriate examinations. Retrieving previous DMIE before deciding to request a new examination is best practice, preventing repeating investigations which have already been performed and providing the necessary information on the X-ray request form. The quality of content and completeness of the request form by the RMPs is essential when determining the type of imaging examination and the associated imaging series conducted. Suboptimal quality like inadequately filled request forms may lead to risking the patient or compromising patient safety like an incorrect or inappropriate examination.

Self-presentation: a cause of unnecessary medical exposures is the self-presentation of patients, who appeal to have a DMIE undertaken. Patients sometimes demand imaging procedures because they have read or heard about them, or because they have discovered information about them in electronic media, including the Internet. They may have received imaging services in the past and believe they should receive them again for the same or new symptoms. Most patients incur little financial liability for imaging services and may interpret the reluctance of a physician to provide them as the withholding of procedures that they are entitled to. Many patients have little understanding of the actual benefits of DMIE, the associated financial costs, and radiation dose (31, 32). Patients may only be referred for DMIE if the MPs are satisfied with the need for such a procedure after the clinical evaluation. Although physicians have a responsibility to contribute to the education of patients, the current payment system discourages physicians from taking time to fulfil this responsibility (31).

Repeat examinations: the fundamental question is, is a repeat justified and must it fully reproduce the original? There is no one size fits all solution; an evidence-based professional judgement must be made. It is important to keep the quality of the DMIE the same as the initial examination.

The reality is, for example, controversial routine repeat head CT in medically managed patients with head injury where the patient's condition may have deteriorated between their first and the follow-up repeat examination. Another factor could be because of a breakdown in communication between the involved HCP and a patient who is not probed during the medical consultation or even in the DMI section where medical imaging providers do not effectively engage with the patient.

Also, a repeat DMIE should not be confused with a poor-quality DMIE, that is, DMIHCP incompetency, suboptimal projections, an incomplete examination, or using a suboptimal imaging protocol. As stated previously could be influenced by the This is quality of information and interpretation of the request order. Including as aspects of considerations of appropriate application of imaging protocols and projections where applicable.

It is important to inform the patient of the reason for the repeat examination because the harms reflect failures in respecting the patient's dignity and autonomy, doing unnecessary and probable harm; injustice through the poor use of DMI resources; the absence of prudence in radiologic thinking; dishonesty through possible inadequate communication with the patient and staff; and a lack of solidarity with the wider community which may need the resources unwisely used. These problems can be resolved through thoughtful multidisciplinary approaches to appropriate protocol development and technical implementation.

It is important to have in the quality assurance component the criteria for acceptable radiographic images and appropriate imaging protocols to ensure that DMIE are complete.

The equipment and its accessories are quality assured through an effective quality control programme in place. It is necessary to have guidelines to make a professional judgement based on DMIHCP competency and the ability to conduct an optimal study. By accessing previous DMIE records, the picture archiving system has partially overcome this challenge. A distributed patient-centric image management system is used (33). From a technological perspective within a digital context, having integrated national health information technology is important. This would enhance the ethical positions of the professions involved and save resources (34).

In this regard DMIHCPs could play an important role in building quality imaging biobanks, the databases that feed the AIs, and the development of national systems that collect and manage these repositories (15). AI can be developed to personalize imaging protocols for modalities such as CT, MRI, and molecular imaging. There is a possibility of using synthetic contrast enhancement, thereby embracing the ethos of personalized and individualized healthcare. Image acquisition by selecting the correct imaging protocol based on patient presentation, clinical question, and region of interest is an important radiographer responsibility which could be automatable.

AI could have a role in automated quality assurance and offer indications for the repeat of an examination in the event of an equivocal or poor-quality image. To achieve an outcome, it is essential that clear protocols are developed to support the implementation of new systems, and where possible quality standards are developed jointly by professionals within DMI and radiotherapy services to support the consistent implementation of proven technologies to high standards. However, the dilemma is these protocols may vary from practice to practice.

Screening and its complexities: it is not unusual to request DMIE for screening purposes. In this section three common screening DMIEs are discussed, that is, chest radiography, mammography, and whole-body CT.

Chest radiographic screening remains a controversial issue and a point of debate with evidence for as well as against it. The amount of radiation a patient is exposed to, during a chest radiograph, is low (0.02 mSv); considering such a low-yield rate, this is minimal for most individuals. If many individuals nationally are being exposed, it would add significantly to the community radiation, cost involved, and time (35). One could use an evidence-based practice approach like pre-employment chest radiographs restricted to symptomatic individuals. The value of the preadmission/employment chest radiograph in a high tuberculosis prevalence country should be assessed, especially for people with occupational exposure to tuberculosis. Added value lies in evaluating the potential health risks to the patients who seek care in the healthcare centre and to the employees. Jasper et al. compared the findings on chest radiographic images in both pre-echocardiography (EG) and post-EG groups and found that among the other abnormalities on chest radiographs in both cohorts, cardiac disease was more commonly seen in the pre-EG group, and lung parenchyma and mediastinal disease were more common in the post-EG group. In the pre-EG group, the assumption was that some participants (depending on the background and socioeconomic status) were for the first time undergoing a detailed complete health screening, and therefore there was a higher number of cardiac abnormalities detected in this group. The expertise of the clinician examining the candidate may vary, and the chest radiograph could alert the clinician to a cardiac abnormality that could have been missed. In the post-EG group, the screening was more effective, picking up tuberculosis which could pose a serious hazard to the patients and other healthcare personnel in the hospital (36). Recently Borkowski and others utilized a readily available, commercial platform to demonstrate the potential of AI to assist in the successful diagnosis of COVID-19 pneumonia on chest radiographic images with a potential impact on future world health crises such as COVID-19 (21). These findings have implications for screening and triage, initial diagnosis, monitoring disease progression, and identifying patients at increased risk of morbidity and mortality. A website was created to demonstrate how such technologies could be shared and distributed to others to combat entities such as COVID-19 moving forward. Further not only did these authors highlight AI in the emergency of a pandemic, but the importance of reliable national guidance is essential for an efficient and coordinated nationwide response and if inadequate then investigate the justification of their actions, and the medico-legal consequences and ethical considerations of deviating from them (37).

Another contentious issue is lung low-dose CT (LDCT) screening. Evidence from large randomized controlled trials (RCTs) shows that LDCT screening for lung cancer reduces lung cancer mortality and can also be cost-effective if stringent risk-based eligibility criteria are employed. A longitudinal RCT, Nederlands–Leuvens Longkanker Screenings Onderzoek (NELSON RCT), found that LDCT screening for lung cancer decreased lung cancer mortality by 24% in high-risk men and 33% in high-risk women over a ten-year period. As the evidence base for LDCT lung cancer screening evolves with improvements to the screening protocols, so do the likely impacts and cost-effectiveness of such a programme. However, the cost-effectiveness of LDCT lung cancer screening varies (38). However, a considerable group of high-risk patients benefits from annual lung cancer CT screening (39).

The benefit and potential harm of LDCT lung cancer screening are fundamentally linked to the individual profiles concerning, on the one hand, the probability of developing lung cancer and, on the other hand, the susceptibility to the cancerogenic effects of ionizing radiations. Accordingly, a greater risk of lung cancer is associated with smoking history and age and additional factors such as asbestos exposure, while the role of gender in modifying the risk is probable but currently undefined. The risk of radiation-induced cancer is inversely proportional to the age at exposure and is greater for women. When considering age, smoking history, and gender on the risk-benefit estimates of lung cancer mortality reduction associated with LDCT screening the harm of cancer development may outweigh the benefit of lung cancer detection in case of young (below 55 years of age) non-smokers, especially if women. This fully justifies efforts in the *a priori* identification of the subjects who are likely to benefit from LDCT through risk prediction modelling and of subjects to whom screening should not be offered. An avenue could involve refining the definition of the high-risk population appropriately. Aside from age and cigarette smoking, which are only two factors, genetic susceptibility variants of lung cancer from genome-wide association studies may be significant in building risk stratification models in the future (40).

The number of false positives is also crucial since it has been demonstrated that 9.2–51% of positive controls at the first round turn out to be false positive which becomes 21% at the second round and 33% at the third round determining 2.3% of minor and 2.73% of major invasive procedures. In approximately 50% of the screened patients an incidental finding is detected which is clinically significant. The average dose exposure reported in large screening trials for a single LDCT ranges between 0.61 and 1.5 mSv, and it increases by 4 mSv if a PET-CT is acquired. Thus, the cumulative risk of cancer incidence, attributable to radiation exposure, according to the BEIR VII report, after ten years of CT screening, is 0.05%. Since the effect of screening on lung cancer mortality has been estimated to be about 5%, the risk of radiation-induced cancer can be considered acceptable (41).

This brings us to the next topic of whole-body CT (WBCT) in the treatment of multiply injured patients, which is beneficial in improving outcomes and therefore part of standard protocol and MI referral guidelines and a valued tool in the justification and for workup in these patients (42). The World Health Organization estimates that radiation dose could be reduced by 30% by applying referral criteria (43). Once referral guidelines are in place, audits may be used for monitoring the use of and compliance with such tools (44). For many patients, there is no controversy as to whether WBCT should be included as part of their management, and most imaging has an MI proforma with specific requesting criteria, to ensure that the examination is justified. However, there is a seemingly increasing number of patients who appear to fulfil these criteria for WBCT, but who turn out to be normal with no trauma-related pathology (21, 42). This is of course highly useful in managing the patient, but the justification for scans in these patients becomes a more complicated issue. WBCT on an average exposes each patient to >20 millisieverts (mSv) of effective radiation dose which increases the risk of cancer mortality to 1 in 900 with a radiation dose of 24 mSv in 35-year-old males and 1 in 1,250 with a radiation dose of 10–20 mSv in the average 45-year-old adult patient. Keeping these statistics in perspective, it becomes the responsibility of the medical fraternity to limit the use of WBCT in polytrauma patients, and proper guidelines regarding the same need to be established.

Another reason for this increase in CT examinations could be attributed to medical insurance programmes reimbursing DMIE. In the private sector in 68% of WBCT screening cases asymptomatic abnormalities called incidentalomas were detected. The most common ones are lung nodules. These non-symptomatic findings result in negative psychological effects on the patient. It is reported that the risk of death for a liver biopsy performed for the purpose of investigating an incidentaloma (from about 1–2 per 1,000 to 4) is the same magnitude as the probability of a deadly tumour.

In CT an important aspect concerns the detection of anomalies affecting venous circulation and their possible consequences at the pulmonary level. In fact, the prevalence of pulmonary embolism is significantly influenced by the diagnostic tests performed, while from a clinical point of view, few patients with venous thrombosis of the lower limbs have respiratory disorders. Although CT increases the micro pulmonary embolism detection rate, it also entails the risk of CA injection, radiation exposure, and increased costs.

The estimation of overdiagnosis in emergency imaging is extremely difficult to evaluate. Even more complex is to determine its impact on radiation exposure, which should be considered proportional to the increase in unjustified imaging examinations (20). In practice, searching for reasonableness and tolerability is a permanent effort directed at acting wisely, based on accumulated knowledge, ethical values, and experiences. Careful and adequate communication with and empathy for the patient, and involving the patient her/himself in the decision-making process can be of help in making the best choice for the patient's well-being (20). The concept of dose tracking can provide useful features in identifying issues of wider interest to patient safety as envisaged originally rather than getting deterred by apprehension of its use and stopping a needed examination. A drive towards patient-specific care is needed (45). The dilemma is that there are several dose monitoring systems that provide an estimation of organ and effective doses, but only a few reports on the validation or assessment of uncertainties and inaccuracies. There is a paucity of information to infer those inaccuracies in effective dose estimations may be larger than one usually encounters in other fields such as the monitoring of critical parameters like blood pressure and blood glucose, more so at the level of doses discussed. There is a need, however, to vet the accuracy of dose estimates provided by these dose monitoring systems (25).

There is also a plethora of AI-driven dose reduction and optimization methods for mammography, CT, PET/CT, and MR time reduction, creating opportunities for faster image acquisition and greater patient throughput. Closing this workforce gap could enable DMISPs more face-to-face interaction with patients and engagement in multidisciplinary meetings, interventional procedures, verification of reports, education, policy-making, and complex clinical decision-making tasks and alleviate fatigue (15). Early research also demonstrates promise in synthetic modality transfer, that is the creation of a CT image from an MRI scan or vice versa, obviating the need for a second imaging procedure entirely. From an ethical perspective the plea is for DMIHCP to simultaneously maintain the core professional value of patient care.

Mammographic screening is used for the early detection of breast cancer in many countries. A main unifying thread is that effective cancer screening must be followed by a decrease in the burden of advanced cancers. The evidence shows that screening mammography has had no or only a limited influence on the burden of advanced breast cancer, and the burden of metastatic breast cancers at diagnosis (46). These authors suggest that the natural history of the condition, including development from latent to declared disease, should be adequately understood before envisioning screening as an option for controlling the mortality caused by a disease. Additionally, false-positive recalls, unnecessary biopsies, and overdiagnosis remain unaffected by improved patient management; the balance in harms and benefits of screening will further deteriorate with the increasing efficacy of therapies (20). Like ductal carcinoma in situ, a rare tumour (less than 5% of the annual incidence of breast cancers) which progresses to invasive carcinoma over a 5 and 15 year interval according to the grade. The estimation of this phenomenon is extremely difficult as demonstrated by a wide range of rates from 0 to 30% (20). With a mean glandular dose for screening mammography, it is between 3 and 10 mGy, influenced by the number of projections acquired, the technology, and patient-related factors (20).

Policy makers implementing affordable and equitable national cancer control plans need to be aware of the serious shortcomings of the evidence base that is often presented to them as beyond doubt. Justifying the continuation of screening mammography is not a question of just taking a pill, but of the threat of lifetime harm due to mutilation, over-treatment, and psychological distress for no gain in the risk of breast cancer death (46).

Additionally, mammographic screening information material has been criticized for ignoring harms and making unwarranted bold claims about insufficient and unbalanced benefits. Given the history and controversies of mammographic screening, the five specific, analyzed, and justified principles may be of practical value in handling the challenges with informing about mammographic screening (47). The suggested five guiding principles are:

- Facts should be presented in ways that acknowledge variation and uncertainties, e.g., by presenting outcomes in ranges.
- The content and the form of information should be developed through open and transparent processes with strong stakeholder involvement.
- Information should be layered.
- Information should be balanced without attempts to frame it.
- Attending mammographic screening should be as easy as not attending.

For many women, autonomous and informed decision-making is not an available option in the breast screening context which positions screening as the "correct" breast health behaviour. An informed choice is made with autonomy, and with an accurate understanding of benefits and harms. The reality is not all patients are dissatisfied with their decisions, despite limited understanding of benefits/harms. These instances create ethical complexities: should such a situation be viewed as acceptable compliance, the desirable exercise of women's autonomy, or as a failed attempt at engaging and supporting women within informed choice processes? These instances perhaps draw attention to the limits of an informed choice (48).

Medical Imaging Contrast Agent Considerations and Safety Issues

There are several different forms of imaging contrast agents (gas, liquid, suspension) (see Figure 1.2) allowing for delivery by mouth, per rectum, intra-luminal, or intravenous/intra-arterial routes. Each different delivery mode has unique applications, for example, an oral contrast agent, a suspension of barium, is used for gastrointestinal studies. Particulate suspensions of barium can only be administered into the intestinal tract. Iodine-based contrast agents can be divided according to osmolarity (high, low, or iso-), ionicity (ionic or non-ionic), and the number of benzene rings (monomer or dimer). Non-ionic contrast agents (CA) cause less discomfort and fewer adverse reactions compared with ionic agents (49).

Double contrast examinations refer to imaging with the positive CA of barium sulphate (rarely water-soluble iodinated) as well as with the negative CA of gas (CO_2 preferable). An exam with only a positive CA is called a single contrast barium enema.

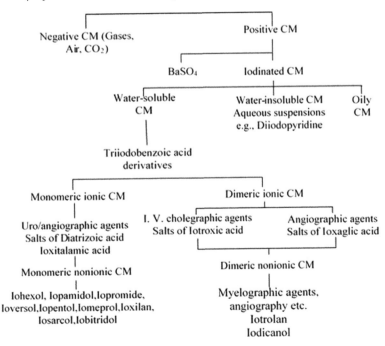

Figure 1.2 An example of medical imaging contrast agent classification (50).

However, the clinical use of these CAs does not come without inherent risk, the most important of which is contrast-induced nephropathy (CIN) (51). Choosing contrast agents, whether it be a prescription for prevention, diagnosis, treatment, or rehabilitation, is a direct, specific, exclusive, and non-delegable responsibility of the MP, thereby demonstrating autonomy and responsibility (52). This includes the verification of indications, contraindications, interactions, and unpredictable individual reactions (see Figure 1.3).

This is dependent on the patient characteristics: anamnesis is necessary to identify risk factors (allergies and kidney disease), clinical conditions and comorbidity (cancer, heart disease, diabetes), age (elderly and children), and physical constitution (body weight). Cofactors include the type of examination, and the technology available can affect the choice of CA to obtain the highest level of diagnostic quality, the minimum impact on higher-risk patients, the optimization of used volumes, and the optimization of injection flows (52). The chemical and physical and symmetry parameters of the CA must be considered for their effectiveness as well as the associated risks. Precautions must be taken, and there is the possibility as well of adverse reactions. One must have knowledge on pharmacokinetic data, preparation, clinical-therapeutic indications, and effects on circulation, permeability, and haemodynamic to determine the appropriateness of CA. This goes hand in hand with several factors, such as the type of examination, the imaging protocol based on the clinical question, the technical characteristics of the equipment, and its configuration.

On this ethical basis, like all MPs, radiologists should also maintain their autonomy in the selection and administration of contrast agents, and any solution to the detriment of this

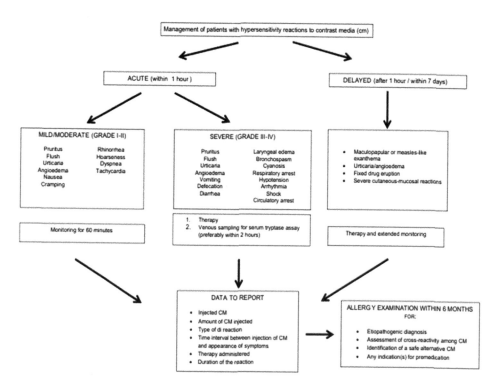

Figure 1.3 Management of patients with hypersensitivity reactions to contrast agents (53, P2).

principle of autonomy is not practicable, including cost-saving. Moreover, limitations in the choice of CA, based on the criterion of the lowest price, might constitute a profile of criminal and civil responsibility (52). Of priority is the effectiveness, safety, and appropriateness in achieving the best outcomes for the patient.

Medical Imaging Errors and Safe Practice Culture

According to Brady, the meaning of the terms "error" and "discrepancy" and the relationship to medical negligence are frequently misunderstood (54). In most cases, DMI interpretation is heavily influenced by the clinical circumstances of the patient, relevant history and previous imaging, and myriad other factors, including biases of which we may not be aware. DMIEs don't come with inbuilt labels denoting the most significant abnormalities, and interpreting them is not a binary process (normal vs abnormal, cancer vs "all-clear").

Diagnostic errors like missing fractures by both DMIHCPs and other HCPs are common, leading to cause for litigation. The attributed reasons are crowding at the emergency department (ED) during early evening hours, a higher threshold for consulting the attending radiologist, and junior MPs releasing patients from the ED without review of the radiographic images by the supervising emergency physician together with clinical findings. In some instances, patients with a clinical suspicion of a scaphoid fracture received a cast. A common missed fracture or doubt occurs with paediatric elbow injuries and imaging thereof. To reduce radiographic errors by ED MPs, a routinely obtained comparison radiograph of the asymptomatic elbow region could be performed. Also, failure to radiograph at the first visit because there was no clinical indication for DMIE is common. Another reason could be due to employing a "wait and see" policy (55). The reality is that often the RMP referrer is frequently required to make patient treatment decisions prior to the availability of the "gold standard" radiology report. Existing evidence has raised concerns regarding the inexperience of some RMPs in interpreting X-rays, increasing the potential for inaccurate or incomplete patient management, which is a concern for patient safety.

Errors in DMI itself: this involves staff shortages and/or excess workload, staff inexperience, inadequate equipment, a less than optimal reporting environment (e.g., poor lighting conditions), or inattention due to the constant repetition of similar tasks and disruptions. Inadequate clinical information or inappropriate expectations of the capabilities of a DMI technique can lead to misunderstanding or miscommunication between the RMP and DMISP (54). With regard to referral request, radiological report and image interpretation, occurring in 4% of DMIE, but are of minor importance. These could include missing a radiographic diagnosis which could lead to an error in diagnosis or complications during interventional procedures and disregard for protocols and rules, or inadequate communication of a DMIHCP with a patient or with RMPs and the lack of recommendation for additional imaging. Postponing or cancelling the interventional procedure may occur, as well as failure to obtain informed consent from the patient and difficulty in the diagnosis in screening mammography. Of this, 30% were convicted in civil proceedings, and 5.5% were convicted in criminal proceedings. There has been a significant increase in the number of court proceedings due to medical error in DMI (56).

Ensuring that the correct examination (e.g., correct procedure, site, test) is performed on the correct patient prevents unnecessary radiation and delayed diagnosis but also prevents a loss of patient trust in the institution and department. However, it is difficult to quantify how often these errors occur, possibly due to underreporting (57).

Errors occur either when a RMP mistakes the sides of the body or when a DMHCP makes labelling errors resulting in wrong-site surgery or misidentification of the side or sites of pathology in radiology reports, compromising patient safety and possibly resulting in morbidity and mortality during imaging-guided procedures. Medication errors in the DMI department are likely to harm patients because of the lack of access to medical documents, impaired patient cognition, lack of familiarity of the DMISP with equipment, and time pressures which create a high-risk scenario. Medication errors in DMI are related to improper doses, using the wrong drug, and drug or dose omission. Errors occur with drugs not used exclusively in DMI—for example, failing to restart an insulin pump in a patient for several hours. Medication-related (including CA) errors certainly occur in the DMI department and are likely underreported.

In relation to patient monitoring, challenges occur when attempting to maintain patient surveillance during DMIE such as limited monitor visibility, lack of familiarity with patients, and the likelihood that patients receiving imaging are in a more acute phase of their illness. During patient transfer to imaging tables, there is the potential for catheters and endotracheal tubes to become dislodged. Additionally, technique-related error, poor image quality, and suboptimal technique contribute to interpretative and diagnostic errors (58).

Further, imaging by MRI or CT scan could become necessary; this will depend on the clinical evaluation and interpretation of the radiographic projections. These practices need to be carefully weighed in terms of the risk versus harm, costs, and value in terms of the management and treatment strategy. The complexity arises when there is discrepancy regarding anatomical regions where fractures are likely to be missed which can lead to major clinical impact such as surgical intervention.

The mediating role of the radiographer: within DMI patients (except for notable subsets, such as mammographers and interventional radiologists), a lack of compensated structured time and space for communication with patients, the permanence and accessibility of radiographic images providing an enduring liability focus, and the natural subjectivity inherent to DMI. Radiographic image interpretation is subject to considerable outcome and hindsight bias, which may complicate the determination of reasonable thresholds for disclosure, apologies, and compensation. Consequently, the determination of whether a radiologic interpretive error has occurred is increasingly a matter of retrospective peer or expert consensus rather than a matter of one expert's opinion. Further, some errors are immediately recognized, and others may not be apparent for an extended period. Additionally, errors may be as a result of a variable and complex interplay of image misinterpretation, procedural mishaps, system processes, and communication lapses (58).

Brown et al.'s study shows that radiographer preliminary image evaluation service was consistent whilst maintaining a reasonably high diagnostic accuracy (59). This form of image interpretation can complement an RMP's diagnosis when a radiologist's report is unavailable at the time of patient treatment (58). Radiographers can play a valuable role in helping rural doctors to correctly interpret radiographic images. Within the interprofessional collaborative practice context this role could be valued in terms of bridging the timely DMI outcomes gap. The dilemma is radiographers are not allowed to diagnose. Though radiographic image interpretation is intricately linked to diagnosis, radiographers are educated and trained in identifying and describing pathology on radiographs; this unequal power relationship may cause those positioned at the base of the hierarchical pyramid, such as radiographers, to remain silent (60).

Error disclosure to patients and its dynamics with data management: within a whole person-centred care context there is an increased emphasis on individual autonomy and consequential acknowledgement of personal preference-driven decision-making. Person centredness is a core dimension of high-quality healthcare, and it expressly includes a person's ability to make well-informed decisions after an error has occurred. Within DMI, although error disclosure has not been explicitly or openly endorsed at the professional societal level, this represents a gap given the strong evidence that patients expect to be informed when errors occur and supportive evidence that event disclosure may be associated with enhanced patient perceptions of quality. A deny and defensive approach rather than open communication hampers transparency and causes possible harm to patients (58). Patients are more likely to sue if they believe they have been dealt with dishonestly and undermining patient autonomy. Transparent communication with patients and families about unanticipated adverse outcomes, proactive explanations, apologies, and—when appropriate—compensation offers is encouraged. It is also recognized that optimal outcomes require a multitiered comprehensive institutional commitment. The shift is to move away from financial benefits and towards beneficial implications for patient safety. The focus is on how institutional cultures react to errors internally.

Although commendable, the variable character of these apology and disclosure laws creates uneven and sometimes weak protections. The laws may protect statements of sympathy but permit the admissibility of statements of responsibility, might unintentionally discourage open disclosure and apology. As a result of an unfortunate confluence of the actions of multiple agents, systems, and processes. To rectify this, a Just Culture philosophy is encouraged, by which good intent is not blamed and MPs are not punished for actions consistent with their training and experience. Such cultures acknowledge personal and systemic accountability for suboptimal performance and use a sophisticated understanding of missed opportunities to improve performance through nonpunitive educational interventions and coaching. To incorporate error disclosure processes into the overall organizational structure, strategies such as the "care for the caregiver" mechanisms can be used, incorporating multiple layers of support, including local departments and units, institutional resources, and external referral networks of psychosocial professionals, such as chaplains, psychologists, and social workers. This can be enhanced through promoting confidence that systems will treat staff with compassion and respect under adverse circumstances. Despite this, many states, insurers, and provider systems steadfastly adhere to the existing tort-based paradigm (58).

AI—who will be responsible for errors?: the primary duty of an MP is to "do no harm", and to continue this virtue, AI must be validated to be safe, accurate, and infallible before being used autonomously. With automation, clarity around the legal implications for inappropriate clinical outcomes should be accounted for as there are multiple stakeholders. The question is who will be liable if AI wrongly reports. To overcome this challenge of learning from medical errors, a root-cause analysis system should be used with transparent application to outcomes that are incorrect, biased, or discriminatory against population subsets (60). Any errors determined to involve AI systems would need to be fed-back to engineers who would in turn complete the feedback loop by ensuring that appropriate adjustments have been made, using technology that allows specific points in the decision-making process to be delineated. There errors must be logged into a national database to determine any large-scale pattern. This would create an AI-related medical errors financial pool, where pre-defined compensation is established for varying levels of medical errors. When errors happen, establishments must always comply with the duty of candour. This approach will enable an improvement in the overall quality of the partnership with AI. It cannot be achieved through a siloed approach; a multidisciplinary AI team should involve MPs, data scientists, and ML engineers. Both industry and the national health system must incorporate the aforementioned from the outset with renewal of policy whenever there is a paradigm shift in AI technology. Roles specific to unsupervised AI and AI augmenting must be outlined. Responsibility appointed to the individuals using AI must be fair and justified and renewed as required (3).

Complexities around data usage: the value of data is defined by the intended usage. There is a difference between owning raw data and processed complex data. Processed data value lies in profit from sharing, reprocessing, further development, and implementing AI in practice—and more importantly dictating how safety and clinical efficacy is integrated. Who owns data at different stages after they have been processed must explicitly be stated, the purpose of the data usage and statement of accountable safe use of the data. It is important that DMIHCPs actively engage in ML development and integration as data scientists and consultants to supervise training and feedback. Projects that target the most clinically relevant and AI systems approval process under the regulatory authority must be transparent regarding data limitations, outcomes, supervision, and validation. To actively integrate AI in the DMI department and to also augment practice and reduce workflow crisis, roles such as medical data scientists and clinical consultants should be included. The NHS and industry must agree upon ownership of AI algorithms and data at different stages of AI use—allowing accountability for a clinically efficient and safe integration (61).

Issues of Occupational Exposure and Safe Practice

The system of radiation protection deals with exposure to radiation in three classes: occupational, medical, and public. Occupational exposures are incurred at work and because of operations within a workplace but may include natural radiation when so specified by the appropriate authority. General principles of optimization should always be borne in mind in the day-to-day administration of radiation protection procedures. Optimization should be employed in determining the most appropriate radiation protection strategies for controlling exposure. Both actual and potential exposures should be considered. The inclusion of potential exposure in optimization assessments should be made a requirement when practical guidance on appropriate techniques becomes available. In addition, it is recommended that dose constraints are used for appropriate work categories in the design of the working environment. That is, for occupations in which the nature of the work requires only minor exposures to radiation, doses should be restricted by design to be less than some value which is lower than the dose limit and which is determined through experience. While dose limits mark the lower bound of unacceptability, dose constraints promote a level of dose control which should be achievable in a well-managed practice. The number of employees who work in circumstances where it is not possible to adopt a dose constraint in the design of the working environment should be kept as small as practicable.

The separation of employees into those covered by a dose constraint and those few who, of necessity, are not, allows for a basic level of pragmatic optimization: the direction of radiation monitoring and assessment resources into areas where they are most needed. In the operation of a practice, it may be appropriate to use investigation levels corresponding to the dose constraints, or to some fraction of the dose constraints, used in the design.

The exposure of employees indirectly involved in work which requires exposure to radiation should be controlled, where applicable, like that employed for members of the public. This may be achieved by adopting a dose constraint related to the public effective dose limit in the design of the working environment for this category of employees. The basis for the control of occupational exposure is the same for women as for men, except that when a pregnancy is declared by a female employee, the embryo or foetus should be afforded the same level of protection as is required for a member of the public (62). Justification is based on the specific benefits and risks for both the mother and the child (63). The stronger the arguments for a critical situation the easier is the justification; in contrast, a vague suspicion would not justify an important exposure. Policies may differ in different practice settings; the rules must be stated in writing and followed consistently. Once the pregnant worker informs her employer of the pregnancy, the employment conditions for her are adjusted to ensure that the equivalent dose to the foetus does not exceed 1 mSv during the "remainder of the pregnancy" (64).

Though one would expect radiographers to be knowledgeable on occupational exposure, in a recent study, Paolocchi et al. in Italy found that although most radiographers (90%) stated their awareness of radiation protection issues, most underestimated the radiation dose of almost all radiological procedures. About 4–5% of participants, respectively, claimed that pelvis magnetic resonance imaging and abdominal ultrasound exposed patients to radiation (65).

Occupational exposure from interventional X-ray procedures is one of the areas in which increased eye lens exposure may occur. Accurate dosimetry is an important element to investigate the correlation of observed radiation effects with radiation dose, to verify the compliance with regulatory dose limits, and to optimize radiation protection practice. In a recent study a dedicated eye lens dosimeter was used. The practical implementation of monitoring eye lens doses and the use of adequate protective equipment remains a challenge. The use of lead glasses with a good fit to the face, appropriate lateral coverage, and/or ceiling-suspended screens is recommended in workplaces with potential high eye lens doses (66).

Additionally, the COVID-19 pandemic resulted in an expectation of a surge in chest imaging which added an additional layer of ethical dilemma. There was a need to consider both the risk of infection and radiation safety (54). These authors attempted a technique through glass to conduct a chest radiograph while taking into consideration the radiation safety and image quality in mobile settings. Image quality was found to be acceptable or borderline in 90% of the images taken through glass, and the average patient dose was 0.02 millisieverts (mSv) per image. The majority (67%) of images were acquired at 110 kV, with an average 5.5 mAs and with source to image distance (SID) ranging from 180 to 300 cm. With staff positioned at greater than 1 m from the patient and at more than 1 m laterally from the tube head outside the room to minimize scatter exposure, air kerma values did not exceed 0.5 microgray (µGy) per image. This method has been implemented successfully (54).

In the Best Interest of the Patients

No doubt DMI has produced undisputable benefits to patients in terms of life expectancy and quality of life (19). However, one cannot ignore the individual as the person. Personhood includes aspects of autonomy, consciousness, memory, selfhood, and personal identity. Ignoring the personhood of the patient could result in a negative experience.

Issues of depersonalization: research findings indicate that patients would not like to be treated as objects. Also, vulnerability is not confined to the aged or disabled but relates to every patient as an individual; hence, one deals with a diverse set of individuals.

In the AI context a perception of depersonalization may arise because the patient feels like just a number and not a person worthy of human interaction. There is a likelihood that AI builds its own values (3). It goes without saying that this powerful technology creates a novel set of ethical challenges that must be identified and mitigated since it could lead to compromising patient preference, safety, privacy, and confidentiality, informed consent, and issues around patient autonomy. Although it ought to be self-evident that AI should not be given any autonomous power to deceive, harm, destroy, or diminish the rights of individual human beings or communities, it may not be possible to programme such ethical principles directly, since the machine is equipped only with pauci-dimensional linguistic and logical-mathematical intelligence. While AI is less subject to cognitive biases experienced by human operators, it is still vulnerable to non-apparent biases in the data and/or algorithm. This also poses the challenge of the "black box" nature of AI systems, which requires a serious and focused effort by those engineering these systems to increase the transparency and expandability of the processes contained within diagnostic or predictive models. Crucially, with life-critical investigations, AI interpretation should require mandatory supervision by a human expert "in-the-loop" to guarantee safety, accountability, and legal liability, in this case, the radiologist. Systemic entry barriers for early innovations in digital health innovation need also to be addressed. A potential national initiative to address such barriers is a sandbox environment that allows patients and HCPs to benefit from early access to new healthcare models, without the high costs associated with large-scale implementation.

Patient data and issues of anonymity and confidentiality: one of the many aspects to consider during the initiation of a referral for an ionizing or non-ionizing DMIE procedure is the patient data such as patient disease characteristics, anatomy, and the nature of lesions, as well as weight, height, age, sex, and gender. Whilst names, date-of-births, and patient ID numbers may not aid much, such as age, gender, ethnicity, and comorbidities may help interpret a person's imaging. Inputting the patient's surname may indicate ethnicity to the algorithm, and this could aid better diagnostic accuracy for the specific patient-group. AI may benefit from taking revealed genetic and environmental factors into the DL algorithm, but equally has the risk of inherent bias and confidentiality breach. For a "fully informed" medical prediction system, some believe that outcomes need to be linked back to a patient's history. This would allow an unrivalled test of technology but can only be achieved with pseudonymization or non-anonymization. This type of data usage can be approved under specific regulations if clear benefits of the data and results are expected.

Another issue is that imaging data from head and face CT scans may also be reconstructed to produce surface rendered images which, if fed into facial recognition software, can distinguish individuals. To safeguard from this, data holders need strong cyber security including an audit trail: transparent, immutable, and verifiable systems, where data accessed at any single instance can be traced and are invulnerable to retrospective manipulation.

Blockchain technology could provide an answer to this level of data confidentiality. As the younger "digitally aware" generation freely shares health data across social media, the tolerance of current risks and meaning of privacy will inevitably evolve. One should always keep in mind patients' best interests and comply with the Caldicott principle of the duty to share information being as important as the duty to protect patient confidentiality (see Figure 1.4).

Building an inclusive system: AI technology has recently been scrutinized for failing to incorporate diversity into its training. Notably, cases of facial recognition not differentiating Chinese faces and African names being characterized as "unpleasant" have been published. This highlights inherent bias which has been described as the single greatest threat of data-driven technology by the Department of Health and Social Care (DoHSC). The Asilomar principles state that AI must "benefit and empower" all of humanity. There are examples of this benevolent practice such as publicly available datasets on bone and chest radiographic images. This sharing mindset is essential for breeding competition amongst companies to catapult AI technology so that it can be most beneficial for MPs in the future. Additionally, a policy gap governing the protection of patient photographic images as they apply to facial recognition technology could threaten proper informed consent, the reporting of incidental findings, and data security. In this regard, a plea for during the development a thoughtfully designed, high-quality, and clinically validated AI technology, which can serve as a prototypical policy for the medical system (11). It would be appropriate to judiciously, safely, and appropriately harness the AI data to benefit patients (2).

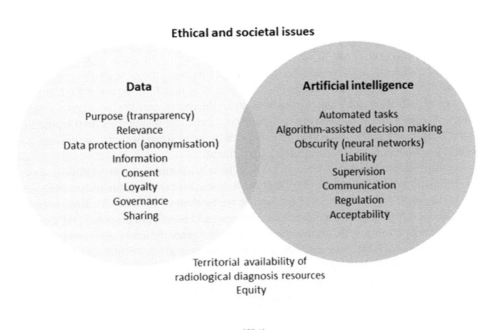

Figure 1.4 Ethical and societal issues raised using big data in healthcare and of artificial intelligence systems in medical imaging (67, P2).

If anonymized data are shared with third parties, a formal explicit consenting process with a "right to be forgotten (data erasure) principle" should be in place. Patient engagement and approval must be obtained before data are made accessible for AI manipulation. Patients need to be empowered with information on their data usage with guidance on how AI works, what problems it will solve (with clearly defined outcomes), when it is used, and if (or when) a human is involved in the decision-making process. It is argued that patient data are used regularly in hospital audits and quality improvement projects without explicit consent because such audits benefit clinical practice and consequently, the patient. The question also arises that once the data are anonymized, how imperative is it to gain explicit consent? For data controllers to utilize data, flow maps must provide legitimate justification for access and data usage. It is necessary to specify the level of anonymization and importantly the data regulations they are implementing. The consenting process should be promoted in the public realm for patients to understand with a focus on equity of access-to-information. A simplified consent form should be easy to understand with "Key Facts" summaries displayed appropriately and an option to opt out. It is important to keep a transparent relationship between the public, industry, and healthcare for AI augmentation (3).

Issues of consent: informed consent is more than simply getting a patient to sign a written consent form; it is a communication process, which requires dedicated time for both the HCP and patient. Applying the principles of informed consent in paediatrics involves consent by the parent/guardian, as well as the consent of a child older than 15 years (25). They are individuals with their own rights of privacy and discretion. Depending on the national legislation, the HCP has a critical role in giving information to and accepting decisions and consent from the right person/s (64). HCP are obliged to include the child in decision-making, according to their maturity and cognitive abilities, and provide the child, as well as the parent/guardian, with a form and amount of information that would be comprehensive and clear. Older children and adolescents, without cognitive deficits, have a right to independently consent. The level of maturity required to provide consent will vary with the nature and complexity of the procedure. In the case of them declining, the HCP is obliged to ask the patient's legal guardian for consent (25). It should be noted that no consent is required in emergency situations if it is impractical to do so. In the case of a medical emergency (where treatment is immediately necessary to save the life of a patient or to prevent serious injury to their health), and the patient is not able to consent to the required treatment at the time, a medical practitioner may perform emergency treatment.

A considerable number of RMPS with DMIE referrals, information sharing stops at explaining the purpose of a DMIE (68). Discussions about expected benefits and possible risks of the paediatric DMIE are less forthcoming, particularly from DMHCPs. RMP would be the more likely to disclose details about the purpose and benefit of a proposed DMIE and the risks of not performing the examination because they generally have a more complete picture of the role of DMI in the patient's care and management, from clinical examination, noted relevant signs and symptoms, and medical history evaluated. Whereas DMPHCPs are more likely to provide details about the DMIE itself including the associated risks because of their expert knowledge in various aspects concerning medical radiation exposure and safety (68). These HCPs need to have the skill on how to provide adequate information to empower patients or their representatives to make informed decisions in giving their consent to matters pertaining to their care or treatment. HCPs should never assume that the patient has already been provided with any information or that the information provided has been fully understood. In this regard, HCPs should take it upon themselves to initiate and engage in a benefit-risk dialogue with patients, to ensure that any needs or concerns of patients or their representatives are appropriately addressed (68).

Consent, restraint, and sedation all pose ethical dilemmas to radiographers. Consent and immobilization are sometimes difficult concepts to explain to people. If there are carers, they play an important role in giving consent and explaining immobilization. For example, radiographers had witnessed people with dementia coming to the imaging department physically restrained to the bed or sedated; however, they agreed that restraint and sedation were a last resort. No radiographers liked using restraints, but some had. There is also a question of putting a person through physical and emotional discomfort, especially where the results of the imaging procedure do not affect the overall healthcare decisions. Radiographers have stated that the justification for the imaging procedure is important and depends on the criticality of the pathology; imaging is used as a tool for ruling out pathologies, and some staff view these imaging procedures as futile (69).

Another example showing that patients are consenting only in the general sense has to do with the age and maintenance of radiologic equipment. Should the patient be informed if the test is done using older equipment that delivers greater doses than newer technology for a similar examination, where the patient could benefit from a significant dose reduction? But even if newer technologies have the potential to minimize the dose of radiation (because they are more efficient and specific in focus), studies have shown that the introduction of digital systems in radiology (a major innovation of the last decade) contributes to an increase in radiation dose (70). Despite its obvious advantages (better diagnostic data, dynamic contrast, pre-/post-processing functionality, electronic transfer, to name but a few), radiographers are largely unaware that digitalization has contributed to overexposure (which can occur without negative effects on image quality in comparison with traditional film-based exams).

HCP-patient relationship: includes principles of mutual responsibility, solidarity, fairness, and tolerance including calling for a just and sound treatment of every person including the provision of honourable working conditions. DMI is a complex encounter which could lead to a conflict or an ethical dilemma. Everyone reacts differently to controlled procedures, and their perspectives may differ from those of well-meaning decision makers (69). During these interactional processes various types of decisions are taken. The presence of the many factors to consider in ethical choice produces a conflict or ethical dilemma, which can be defined as a decision-making problem between two possible moral imperatives, neither of which is unambiguously acceptable or preferable. Dilemmas may arise out of various sources of behaviour or attitude. For instance, dilemmas may arise out of failure of personal character, conflict between personal and professional values, or even between them and those of a particular patient or society (23). Which could result in dealing with multiple aspects of care related issues within an individual patient trajectory.

The mere fact that it has been prescribed by their doctor may impede a patient's ability to properly understand the implications (and the associated risks) of the medical intervention. Once prescribed, the inadequate justification is forgotten and only the imperative for the exam remains. Due to persistent medical and social views of radiology as a service (71), it minimizes the importance of informing and being informed about this risk, thereby jeopardizing the principle of autonomy (i.e., the routine nature of radiology induces a certain tolerance or blindness towards risks). Many aspects of radiology are unknown to patients; for example, the quest for the best quality image (higher level of diagnostic information) with high-dose technologies is an imperative stronger than patient protection (72). By consenting in a general sense to the medical act, the patient is expressing agreement with a procedure, but not to the specifications of the DMIE procedures per se (73).

Patient imaging risks versus harm: when considering the harm versus risk during a referral for a DMIE, practitioners (RMPs) should also consider that various population groups have different radio sensitivity, the unborn foetus being especially highly radiosensitive. The biological effect of radiation depends on the age and tissue of an individual exposed. It could lead to exposing pregnant patients and children to unnecessary medical exposures (24). For example, an adolescent female of childbearing age must be considered as potentially pregnant and should be asked. The ten-day rule must be applied. As the hormone level does not increase before implantation (with individual variation), it is recommended not to perform the test earlier than ten days after ovulation; blood tests are more sensitive and, thus, become positive around two days earlier. This is because the chances of being pregnant up to this time are minimal since fertilization takes place between the 11th and 14th day. However, in case of urgency an examination can be performed under the benefit versus risk consideration. This is supported by posters in the department (63). Dose may be demonstrated, e.g., by using symbols, background radiation, or verbal scales, whereas risks maybe indicated by using verbal or numerical scales. Patients must always have the opportunity to ask questions.

Radiation exposure during the first two weeks after fertilization is believed to result in an "all or nothing" event where either normal development of the foetus ensues, or a spontaneous abortion occurs (63). The biological effect of radiation depends on the age and tissue of an individual exposed. It could lead to exposing pregnant patients and children to unnecessary medical exposures (24). The threshold of foetal dose for inducing a spontaneous abortion is estimated to be 50 to 100 mGy or higher—a greater dose than any single CT should ever reach. However, the background rate of spontaneous abortion is approximately 50% at this particular stage. Teratogenesis is most common between the 2nd and 25th weeks, especially between the 8th and 15th weeks. Deterministic effects exhibit a threshold of around 100 mGy even during the most sensitive phase of organogenesis. Given the rapid development and differentiation of organs during this stage, radiation exposure of more than 50 to 100 mGy to the foetus can cause congenital malformations as well as reduction of IQ, microcephaly, and intrauterine growth restriction. Carcinogenesis relates to the stochastic effect of radiation and has the potential to occur at any dose; hence there is no threshold below which carcinogenesis cannot occur. This risk is minimal with DMIE (27, 63). Although uncertainties exist in estimation, the risk of carcinogenesis may be comparable in the second and third trimesters and part of the first trimester. The lifetime attributable risk of developing cancer is approximately 0.4% per 10 mGy foetal dose. After implantation of the conceptus in utero exposure <100 mGy has no proven deterministic effects, but the stochastic effects of cancer induction, though minimal, are likely to exist and increase in proportion to the dose.

The ALARA principle means that US and MRI and any non-imaging diagnostic examinations should be considered before DMI or NM. When ionizing radiation is appropriate, lower exposure is preferred to higher exposure if imaging quality is high enough to answer the clinical question. The anatomical area exposed to direct radiation is the most important factor predicting the uterine dose. Of utmost importance in a pregnant woman, the clinical risk of not performing the DMIE examination must be evaluated. If the foetus is in the direct beam, the procedure should be tailored to reduce the foetus dose (i.e., for radiographic examinations: collimate the beam, increase kVp, remove the anti-scatter grid; for CT: collimate the beam and reduce the scan to the very specific area of interest). Fluoroscopic time must always be limited to the minimum. Any department offering imaging services, beyond complying with general quality standards, has several duties regarding the radiation exposure of pregnant patients. The duties of a department of radiology, communication and decision include information, screening for pregnancy, counselling, documentation, and the decision on the best justified examination. For example, a mandatory pregnancy test should be conducted for all females of childbearing age undergoing DMIE, or a pregnancy test may be necessary if the patient has missed the monthly menstrual period. Effective communication between the RMP and DMISP may help in reducing unnecessary examinations, as it can iron out issues without subjecting patients to further imaging.

It is important to track the total foetal radiation exposure throughout pregnancy in patients undergoing multiple DMIE and to explain these risks to the gravid patient, and this should be a component of informed consent. The effect on the mother cannot be ignored, as the proliferation of breast glandular tissue throughout pregnancy increases its radio sensitivity and subsequently the risk of breast cancer. There is no risk to lactation due to ionizing radiation from diagnostic studies (63).

The frequency of DMIE requiring radiation exposure in children (especially CT) is rapidly increasing. The risk associated with low doses is estimated to be small, such that it cannot be quantified accurately, as even very large studies would lack adequate statistical power to demonstrate small differences. Further, debate and research are fundamental to progress radio sensitivity in children as an area of science because in children, developing organ mitoses are more frequent, and children have a longer life expectancy in which to express risk. However, cancer incidence does not increase linearly with mutation frequency, and cancer incidence significantly increases in old age with an increased risk of malignancies when immune compromised. It may be hypothesized that low-dose radiation could enhance the immune system response and thus reduce cancer incidence overall (64).

According to Høilund-Carlsen, current rules and limitations on the use of medical low dose ionizing radiation (LDR) are based on a hypothetical model, the linear no threshold (LNT) concept, which has never been proved to be right (74). The result is regulations that are too tight and that limit the development and use of molecular imaging and prevent its potential from being fully unfolded to the benefit of patients and society. Since this serves no-one's interest, the rules need to be changed to facilitate and not complicate the realization of this potential. This excessive restriction is particularly regrettable considering that molecular imaging is about to revolutionize our perception of many of the worst diseases that afflict mankind and to significantly improve their management. Here we argue that LDR is widely inert and should be used for medical imaging more extensively and without restrictions if the effective dose to the patient from a single exposure or the annual cumulated dose from repeat examination stays below 100 mSv, or even 200 mSv (75).

AI learns and implements ever faster and more efficient methods of CT and MR image reconstruction; it is possible to realize abbreviated sequences and improved scanner productivity. At the same time also, it should be noted that patients can have many concurrent medical issues which may not be apparent from written medical records or DMI reports. For example, in interstitial lung disease, even a biopsy result is not necessarily a gold standard, as there can be sampling bias and histological mimics. Hence, the final diagnosis is often the result of a multidisciplinary review of each case with inputs from the primary respiratory physician, surgeon, radiologist, and pathologist, which may not be apparent in the annotation process. Furthermore, in complex cases, independent reads by different radiologists can lead to different assessments on ground truth labels (interobserver variability) (3).

Research is underway to address these challenges by advancing deep learning approaches to learn from images in scenarios where clearly demarcated annotations are unavailable. Approaches such as these require validation, have standards and tools to facilitate and encourage collaborative data use agreements, and address important concerns around patient privacy and data security. There are standards for de-identification, encryption, and network access. Awareness of high-profile data leaks and data security is adequately addressed. There are data integrity standards, grounded in rigorous evaluation of the different approaches for data curation as well as the degree and types of labelling and annotation. The potential research gains must be weighed against the ethical protection of patients' autonomy and rights to privacy, and the responsibilities of clinical institutions to protect the data they contain. Taking into consideration the importance of the AI integration and translational process into existing hospital information and radiology systems, where they can be validated clinically and systemically. This includes addressing questions around whether AI models should reside inside PACS like any other analytical tool or in between image acquisition modality and PACS—presenting numerical opinions to the radiologist in the form of a mini-report such as calcium scoring, bone age, myocardial tissue native relaxation properties, and likelihood ratios. These challenges present important opportunities for research and development.

A collaborative framework is required for HCP and AI technologists and stakeholders to collectively work together to drive progress. There are funding and resource allocations for AI and initiatives developing AI at a broad strategic level and possibilities for research. How does one balance protecting the patient's individual interests and at the same time make sure society benefits? A sensible approach would be to assert that "if big data research of today is clinical practice tomorrow", then this research should be considered a core business of the restructured hospital system. Early adopters must also be prepared to deal with any unintended consequences and failures (conspicuous or otherwise) arising from disruptive technology. The framework to address issues such as the risks of bad actors/hackers compromising AI systems is needed within the vocabulary of institutional review boards (IRBs) and as complementary amendments to ensure ethics, safety, and data protection (2).

Strategies to Consider in Dealing with the Myriads of Dilemma

From an ethical point of view, should the current situation be worrying, and should it raise questions about what constitutes "good clinical practice"? It is also important to add that ethical requirements can be difficult to operationalize. Although ethics considers the challenges present in the professional environment, and confronts them with the principles of bioethics, it is not always able to counter the structural constraints that leave little room for change in practice (73).

The issue is complex insofar as information provision is only one part of an episode of care. However, if a duty to inform were better established in DMI, it could address both the problem of overuse and the lack of information that can be found in current DMI practice. Greater awareness on the part of both professionals and patients about the risks of DMIE would help, to some extent, in countering the problem of overuse. MPs could better exercise their profession in alignment with fundamental ethical principles and the ethics of responsibility, while patients would receive care that preserved their dignity and integrity (73).

General campaigns aimed at the public or all patients with a given disease may be less effective than efforts that target point of care when each specific patient needs to decide whether to have a DMIE performed. Instead of the current typical pre-DMIE conversation, which generally involves a RMP simply notifying the patient that DMIE is ordered, a shared decision-making process requires comprehension of the likely benefits versus the potential detrimental effects of testing, including the detection and investigation of unrelated findings. An informed consent process of that kind may improve transparency and reduce confusion regarding follow-up and treatment options. However, paradoxically, the exposure of patients to information overload and medical jargon may tilt them towards choosing to do more rather than less. This may be an even greater concern if the RMPs go into a multitude of diagnostic tests that are possibly useful and discuss all diagnostic test options. It is unknown what threshold of perceived utility should be used by a physician before opening a conversation with a patient on whether a test should be performed (29).

One must be knowledgeable on how the benefits and risks are weighed and understand the justification principle. On communication, the ICRP recommend RMPs should always inform their patients of the risks from DMIE. To improve communication, fact sheets on DMIE may be provided to the patients bearing the information on the benefits and risks (74). Also, like adherence to preparation instructions, short interviews can be conducted with all patients before examination. Using simple language, DMIHCPs should ask questions that cannot be answered by a yes or no. Using this approach, the patient is encouraged to explain exactly how he or she has prepared for the examination, which may make those with poor adherence more easily identified. When patients need to be given instructions, the teach-back method described can be used to improve comprehension and has been shown to improve adherence to medical instructions (76).

The solution could lie in a better use of what resources are available. This can be accomplished by assessing the role of each HCP, the medical and sociological context, and the role of DMI within medical practice to understand what "doing better" means. To redefine DMI through exploration within the healthcare context by not only focusing on an episodic care based approach but holistically addressing aspects of safety and health and well being. All stakeholders work together with emphasis on culture of safety and culturally safe context (73).

Then in the day-to-day practice effective guidelines and protocols should be in place with a standard approach to follow dose reference levels for each DMIE. For example, in paediatric imaging to reduce exposure of children, interventions such as Image Gently and EuroSafe Imaging could be used (64). For instance, the use of gonadal shielding issues. Like placement of this devise could obscure crucial anatomical structures. The recommendation is not to use shielding at all. Assuming that with proper collimation, added filtration, and technique selection, the gonadal dose without lead shielding from the examination should be 25–50 µGy for boys and 13–25 µGy for girls, the estimated increased risk from omitting gonad shielding is relatively small. This could be enhanced by reducing the number of radiographs, and teaching appropriate collimation technique can be beneficial rather than gonad shield devices (64).

Effective interventions may entail educating the public and concurrent engagement at multiple points within the system involving both HCP and patient to address outcomes that reflect safety and harms. Healthy individuals and patients can be counselled that DMIE not only has associated risks due to radiation and intravenous contrast, but also can lead to the detection of incidental findings. Flowcharts and diagrams can be created to demonstrate the possible scenarios (29). To help both patients and professionals with this challenging issue, digital educational information can be used for patients and separately for RMPs and DMIHCPs. For the public educational materials along with videoclips with information about radiation and different examinations can be displayed on the Internet (the Virtual Hospital 2.0). Develop national or institutional specific compact guidelines defining the content and responsibilities for providing information (77).

Training Issues within the Medical Profession and DMI

The ideal would be a knowledgeable and well-trained student playing an important role in the creation of a positive radiation safety culture. According to Abuelhia, knowledge of the effective doses in radiological imaging using ionizing radiation is very important to avoid adverse biological health effects, and deterministic or stochastic effects associated with overexposure (78). It is a legal obligation for doctors to comply with the ionizing radiation regulations, nationally and internationally, and with basic health and safety standards. Although the knowledge level of the interns concerning effective doses was higher than that of senior medical students, the overall knowledge level was poor. A radiation protection course of 5–10 h should include basic knowledge on patient radiation protection such as the biological effects of radiation, justifications of exposures, procedure optimization, risk-benefit analysis, typical doses for each type of examination, etc. In addition, knowledge of the advantages and disadvantages of the use of ionizing radiation in medicine should be part of radiation protection education and training for medical students (19). The integration of radiation protection and safety topics into medical programmes and the inclusion of such topics during conferences help in improving their knowledge regarding the justification of DMIE (24). Also, residency education on topics such as request orders and justification like answer the following questions: is it necessary? What are the consequences of performing the test? What are the alternative options (indicate the associated benefits and risks)? What is the likely outcome with no further workup (29)?

Image interpretation and evaluation should entail integrating a visual framework. That is, for almost every pathological condition a student needs to learn what could be a radiologic manifestation to contribute to the diagnostic decision-making processes and procedures. For instance, in teaching clinical reasoning—going through the patient's history, generating a differential diagnosis, and deciding which is the best (most accurate and cost-efficient) test to confirm the diagnosis to commence treatment. This will also aid in preparing medical students adequately for clinical practice (79). Interns value the training because they need to arrange and provisionally interpret appropriate DMIE images to provide quality and timely patient care. It could also create an awareness of DMI early in their career encouraging students to develop an interest in, and maybe later apply for, specialty training in radiology (24).

Further DMI teaching requires shared teaching platforms which involve clinicians, anatomists, and DMI field experts because of the high technological sophisticated examinations producing complex images which take DMI field specialists some years to competently interpret and read (79).

In a recent systematic review Chew and others suggest that the merit of DMI teaching in the undergraduate medical curriculum comes with its own complexities and issues. It depends on the curriculum whether the institution adopts a problem-based or conventional medical curriculum. MI is often taught against a backdrop of limited university or departmental support and resources and ongoing increasing clinical workload (79). DMI training was informal and infrequent. Some medical graduates felt under-prepared for their role as clinicians regardless of the teaching they received, the demanding technologically evolving DMI field and insufficient radiologists to deliver safe and effective patient care (24).

However, technological advances mean we can still provide interactive, authentic immersive teaching using a variety of virtual and online tools with limited manpower. Standardized validated web-based self-marking, nationally deployable examinations using exquisite whole-body CT/MRI images of real patients. There is also a shift toward the migration of DMI education into the social media sphere is happening, as well as small group teaching, clinical seminars, case presentations, structured and self-learning, defined learning objectives, assessment in DMI, and flipped classrooms. These serve as platforms for active, experiential, and authentic learning. As Chew and others state, "the right test for the right patient at the right time" (79).

One could make use of DMIE post-processing image manipulation techniques so that the quality and focus of the image are adjusted to the level of clinical suspicion. For instance, a chest CT scan protocol to rule out pulmonary embolism could be modified to have only medium resolution for skeletal tissues and breast (in female patients) and high resolution for the pulmonary vessels. As a result, pulmonary nodules, abnormal marrow signals, and breast irregularities will be less likely to be detected. A similar idea involves the visual projection of only the radiographic fields relevant to the clinical question. Anatomical sites outside the region of clinical concern ("low-yield territories") would be imaged but shadowed on the final image. It might be argued that a limited radiographic image is equivalent to a partial physical examination and that a restricted field jeopardizes the ability to make an accurate unifying diagnosis. This may be true for complicated cases. Although this approach would not reduce the number of initial tests, it could potentially prevent the cascade of tests that follow an incidental finding. Dealing with how this focus may affect the malpractice climate would also be necessary.

DMIHCPs could serve as gate keepers by use of a case-based approach by consulting them on whether the requested examination is justified based on the clinical question at hand. Well-orchestrated strategies are needed that can reduce unnecessary diagnostic imaging. A fundamental question is whether these strategies work and how best to determine whether they do without compromising patient well-being (29).

AI and educational implications: HCP education *should* be reframed away from a focus on knowledge recall to a focus on training students to interact with and manage AI machines. It is suggested that these changes must take place by 2024, and the respective healthcare employers should upskill existing staff to ensure comparative knowledge to support technological adaptation and the necessary changes in work practices and workplace culture. This includes the statistical underpinning of AI systems to assess for AI outputs in the workplace practice domain, and leadership roles will emerge to drive change management processes during the deployment and ongoing maintenance of vendor-specific systems. Education programmes must include automated technology operation, core computer science skills, and technical processes for supervising and assuring automated outputs and actions. It is highly strongly recommended that extensive research evidence is gathered to validate and prove that AI is beneficial to the patient and thereafter implement in clinical practice (80).

It is important that when trialling the implementation of an AI algorithm for the field expert in interpreting AI-guided results and at the same time identify potential ethical dilemmas. For instance, it could be that machine learning algorithms might not provide equally accurate predictions of outcomes across race, gender, or socioeconomic status. For example, in terms of image interpretation, supervised learning algorithms require an enormous collection of DMI data, validated by experts, and widely agreed upon by both the DMIHCP and the computer science community. The limitation is that, despite the validation, the data are only fit for the population from which they are retrieved. Once again despite the praise for its capabilities in terms of work volume and throughput efficiency, AI must not be at the detriment of staff or patient well-being and quality of care (61). For example, AI should maximize the role of the DMIHCPs in improving patient pathways and outcomes through AI-supported image interpretation. It should enable MPs to provide immediate results to patients to facilitate the triage of patients for additional DMIE or direct them to other specialities (81). Creating the educational resources necessary for an AI curriculum will require the collaborative efforts of multiple stakeholders including national and international societies and academic radiology departments (81, 82).

DMI and radiation therapy educational programmes are regularly reviewed to support the development of the appropriate skills within the profession. Demonstrate essential leadership to support, test, and deliver safe systems of work and safely implement them in practice. Embrace, adopt, and adapt technology, ensuring that practice is evidence based and based on the patient. HCPs should use AI as a support tool, an adjunct to, not a replacement for, clinical judgement and professionally accountable decision-making. Develop a broad understanding of how algorithms work prior to implementation in clinical practice, to be aware of the limitations of technology. Ensure that algorithms are used to improve patient experience as well as working conditions for DMIHCP imaging healthcare providers, recognizing the need for multiple outcome measures when determining departmental effectiveness and an awareness of the role that increased imaging volumes may have on patient experience. Work and collaborate with the wider radiographic community, industry, and a multidisciplinary team to be involved in designing, developing, and validating AI for use in clinical practice. Ensure AI solutions are developed to solve current and future MI problems.

AI and regulatory implications: the regulation of AI in healthcare is a complex topic and differs depending on location. As AI increases in influence on healthcare decisions, rules around the decision-making process and legal indemnity (including national frameworks for medical defence companies) need to be modified. A regulatory system should protect both patients and HCPs by defining the professional responsibilities of HCPs using AI and the management of risk associated with AI tools. Whilst we may believe that we live in an informed society, the media doesn't always represent the true nature of AI (3). The national framework for training AI collaborations between industry, academia, and the NHS must share patient data in a symbiotic manner to bring about an overall benevolent outcome for the patient (12). Within a broader theoretical framework, it is important to distinguish between data analysis (in this case, the AI-device output) and decision-making. Based on an evidence-based medicine context, the best external evidence such as data from high-quality studies and meta-analysis and guidelines from governmental bodies and medical societies needs to be integrated with patients' preferences and values and the use of discipline field expert knowledge (22).

The introduction of AI technology into daily practice requires thorough planning with frameworks developed to standardize clinical efficacy, governance, and medico-legal protection. Interfacing and integrating built-in safety developing AI from its current infancy to an automated system in healthcare is an iterative process dotted with growth spurts and disruptive events (60). DMIHCPs have a greater responsibility in advising on, defining, and disclosing the radiation risks associated with DMIEs in line with ionizing radiation regulatory requirements. This may include, but is not limited to, developing best practice guidance on explaining risks of AI-driven systems to patients, ascertaining the influence of AI processes on human interaction and decision-making. Maintain awareness of and lobbying for adaptation to legislation in each country to maximize the benefit of AI to patients and DMIHCPs. Ensure investment in the development of the existing and future workforce through funded professional development (81).

AI and research: research involving AI systems must be conducted in an ethical way, communicating with patients on how their data may be used to develop and test AI. All stakeholders are involved in the piloting and research of algorithms prior to clinical implementation. It is important to have knowledge and understand how algorithms arrive at decisions and probability errors within these decisions to enable the effective communication of findings to patients. Maintain and develop core skills and competencies to act as a sense check to AI-supported clinical decisions (for example scan planning in CT, image interpretation triage). Work at national and international levels with policy makers to ensure that investment in AI research focuses across the scope of practice within imaging and radiotherapy services (81).

The responsible and safe use of AI technology includes making the potential harms related to the use of AI technology transparent to all involved. Proposals should be set up and contribute to populate a large single interoperable repository of health imaging, enabling the development, testing, and validation of AI-based health imaging solutions to improve diagnosis, disease prediction, and follow-up of the most common forms of cancer and chronic diseases (3). Though a global imaging project is underway towards a sustainable imaging infrastructure allowing access to cutting-edge research before DMI data can be fed into ML, it needs to be made "AI ready" and the data need purification. For the data to be fully centralized, digitization is required. Although most radiological imaging exists in this format, the associated reports and patient documentation do not (3).

A recent publication by Allen et al. states, for the healthcare system to become a viable effective pathway for both foundational and translational research, ensuring a reliable deployment of AI in clinical practice is essential (81). Workshops are essential to identify current knowledge and research gaps to identify and prioritize future initiatives for foundational and translational research in AI for medical imaging as illustrated in Figure 1.5.

Based on this conceptual framework both foundational and translational research activities are interconnected. Foundational research leads to new image reconstruction and labelling methods, new machine learning algorithms, and new explanation methods, each of which enhances the datasets, data engineering, and data science leading to the deployment of AI applications in medical imaging.

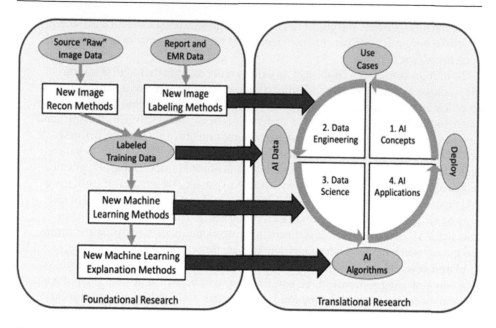

Figure 1.5 A conceptual framework illustrating both foundational and translation research in AI in a DMI context (83, P3).

Conclusion

In conclusion, Liew et al. cite the great diagnostician, Sir William Osler, who declared that "Medicine is a science of uncertainty and an art of probability". He did so in the days when diagnosis depended mainly on clinical history and examination, not on an image (2, P22). Whereas Carlton and Adler call medical imaging "an art and a science", a process to create visual representations of the human body (84). The embodied patient a person lives with uncertainty a fundamental patient experience of illness and disease. Medical images can provide an illusory visual representation of certainty, but patient distress and suffering do not end when a diagnostic label is found. The patient as a person wants reassurance and yearns to return to normality, to a quality-of-life experience of wellness. Building on the ethical, compassionate roots of good medical practice, can AI augment and refine human judgement in the constant pursuit of caring for human wellness?

References

1. Maliborski A, Zegadło A, Placzyńska M, Sopińska M, Lichosik M, Jobs K. The role of modern diagnostic imaging in diagnosing and differentiating kidney diseases in children. *Developmental Period Medicine*. 2018;22(1):81–7.
2. Liew CJ, Krishnaswamy P, Cheng LT, Tan CH, Poh AC, Lim TC. Artificial intelligence and radiology in Singapore: Championing a new age of augmented imaging for unsurpassed patient care. *Annals of the Academy of Medicine of Singapore*. 2019 Jan 1;48(1):16–24.

3. Mudgal KS, Das N. The ethical adoption of artificial intelligence in radiology. *BJR|Open*. 2020;2(1):20190020. doi.org/10.1259/bjro.20190020

4. Matilainen K, Ahonen SM, Kankkunen P, Kangasniemi M. (2017). Radiographers' perceptions of their professional rights in diagnostic radiography: A qualitative interview study. *Scandinavian Journal of Caring Sciences*. 2017;31(1):139–45. doi.org/10.1111/scs.12335

5. Strudwick RM, Day, J. Interprofessional working in diagnostic radiography. *Radiography*. 2014;20(3):235–40. doi.org/10.1016/j.radi.2014.03.009

6. Wiles K, Bahal, N, Engward H, Papanikitas A. Ethics in the interface between multidisciplinary teams: A narrative in stages for inter-professional education. *London Journal of Primary Care*. 2016;8(6):100–4. doi.org/10.1080/17571472.2016.1244892

7. Morley L, Cashell A. Collaboration in health care. *Journal of Medical Imaging and Radiation Sciences*. 2017;48(2):207–16. doi.org/10.1016/j.jmir.2017.02.071

8. Hardy M, Harvey H. Artificial intelligence in diagnostic imaging: Impact on the radiography profession. *The British Journal of Radiology*. 2020;93(1108):20190840. doi.org/10.1259/bjr.20190840

9. Mahmood A, Bang D, Ahmadabadi MN, Bahrami B. (2013). Learning to make collective decisions: The impact of confidence escalation. *PLoS One*. 2013;8(12):e81195. doi.org/10.1371/journal.pone.0081195

10. Makanjee CR, Bergh AM, Hoffmann WA. (2018). Distributed decision making in action: Diagnostic imaging investigations within the bigger picture. *Journal of Medical Radiation Sciences*. 2018;65(1):5–12. doi.org/10.1002/jmrs.250

11. Rigby MJ. Ethical dimensions of using artificial intelligence in health care. *AMA Journal of Ethics*. 2019 Feb 1;21(2):121–4. doi.org/10.1001/amajethics.2019.121

12. Re GL, De Luca R, Muscarneri F, Dorangricchia P., Picone D., Vernuccio F., ... Russo A. Relationship between anxiety level and radiological investigation. Comparison among different diagnostic imaging exams in a prospective single-center study. *La radiologia medica*. 2016;121(10):763–8. doi.org/10.1007/s11547-016-0664-z

13. Lewis S, Heard R, Robinson J, White K, Poulos A. The ethical commitment of Australian radiographers: Does medical dominance create an influence? *Radiography*. 2008 May 1;14(2):90–7. doi.org/10.1016/j.radi.2007.01.004

14. McDougall RJ, Gillam L, Ko D, Holmes I, Delany C. Balancing health worker well-being and duty to care: An ethical approach to staff safety in COVID-19 and beyond. *Journal of Medical Ethics*. 2021 May 1;47(5):318–23.

15. Lewis SJ, Gandomkar Z, Brennan PC. Artificial Intelligence in medical imaging practice: Looking to the future. *Journal of Medical Radiation Sciences*. 2019 Dec;66(4):292–5. doi.org/10.1002/jmrs.369

16. Malone J, Zölzer F. Pragmatic ethical basis for radiation protection in diagnostic radiology. *The British Journal of Radiology*. 2016;89(1059):20150713. doi.org/10.1259/bjr.20150713

17. Kadivar M, Manookian A, Asghari F, Niknafs N, Okazi A, Zarvani A. Ethical and legal aspects of patient's safety: A clinical case report. *Journal of Medical Ethics and History of Medicine*. 2017;10:15.PMID: 30258549

18. Varkey B. Principles of clinical ethics and their application to practice. *Medical Principles and Practice*. 2021;30(1):17–28. doi.org/10.1159/000509119

19. Kada S. (2017). Awareness and knowledge of radiation dose and associated risks among final year medical students in Norway. *Insights into Imaging.* 2017;8(6):599–605. doi. org/10.1007/s13244-017-0569-y

20. Salerno S, Laghi A, Cantone MC, Sartori P, Pinto A, Frija G. Overdiagnosis and over imaging: An ethical issue for radiological protection. *La radiologia medica.* 2019 Aug;124(8):714–20. doi.org/10.1007/s11547-019-01029-5

21. Borkowski AA, Viswanadhan NA, Thomas LB, Guzman RD, Deland LA, Mastorides SM. Using artificial intelligence for COVID-19 chest x-ray diagnosis. *Federal Practitioner.* 2020 Sep;37(9):398. doi.org/10.12788/fp.0045

22. Pesapane F, Volonté C, Codari M, Sardanelli F. Artificial intelligence as a medical device in radiology: Ethical and regulatory issues in Europe and the United States. *Insights into imaging.* 2018 Oct;9(5):745–53. doi.org/10.1007/s13244-018-0645-y

23. Iavicoli S, Valenti A, Gagliardi D, Rantanen J. Ethics and occupational health in the contemporary world of work. *International Journal of Environmental Research and Public Health.* 2018 Aug;15(8):1713. doi.org/10.3390/ijerph15081713

24. Glenn-Cox S, Hird K, Sweetman G, Furness E. Radiology teaching for interns: Experiences, current practice and suggestions for improvement. *Journal of Medical Imaging and Radiation Oncology.* 2019;63(4): 454–60. doi.org/10.1111/1754-9485. 12896

25. Nurković JS, Petković P, Tiosavljević D, Vojinović R. Measurement of bone mineral density in children with cerebral palsy from an ethical issue to a diagnostic necessity. *BioMed Research International.* 2020;2020:7282946. doi.org/10.1155/2020/7282946

26. Ablordeppey EA, Drewry AM, Beyer AB, Theodoro DL, Fowler SA, Fuller BM, Carpenter C R. Diagnostic accuracy of central venous catheter confirmation by bedside ultrasound versus chest radiography in critically ill patients: A systematic review and meta-analysis. *Critical Care Medicine.* 2017;45(4):715–24. doi.org/10.1097/CCM .0000000000002188

27. Armao D, Semelka RC, Elias J Jr. Radiology's ethical responsibility for healthcare reform: Tempering the overutilization of medical imaging and trimming down a heavyweight. *Journal of Magnetic Resonance Imaging.* 2012;35(3):512–7. doi.org/10 .1002/jmri.23530

28. John SD, Moore QT, Herrmann T, Don S, Powers K, Smith SN, Morrison G, Charkot E, Mills TT, Rutz L, Goske MJ. The image gently pediatric digital radiography safety checklist: Tools for improving pediatric radiography. *Journal of the American College of Radiology.* 2013 Oct 1;10(10):781–8.

29. Oren O, Kebebew E, Ioannidis JPA. Curbing unnecessary and wasted diagnostic imaging. *JAMA.* 2019;321(3):245–6. doi.org/10.1001/jama.2018.20295

30. Malone J, Guleria R, Craven C, Horton P, Järvinen H, Mayo J, O'reilly G, Picano E, Remedios D, Le Heron J, Rehani M. Justification of diagnostic medical exposures: Some practical issues. Report of an international atomic energy agency consultation. *The British Journal of Radiology.* 2012 May;85(1013):523–38. doi.org/10.1259/bjr/42893576

31. Hendee WR, Becker GJ, Borgstede JP, Bosma J, Casarella WJ, Erickson BA, Maynard CD, Thrall JH, Wallner PE. Addressing overutilization in medical imaging. *Radiology.* 2010 Oct;257(1):240–5. doi.org/10.1148/radiol.10100063

32. Al-Mallah A, Vaithinathan A G, Al-Sehlawi M, Al-Mannai M. Awareness and knowledge of ionizing radiation risks between prescribed and self-presenting patients for common diagnostic radiological procedures in Bahrain. *Oman Medical Journal.* 2017;32(5):371–7. doi.org/10.5001/omj.2017.72

33. Jabarulla MY, Lee H. Blockchain-based distributed patient-centric image management system. 2020;arXiv preprint arXiv:2003.08054. doi.org/10.3390/app11010196

34. Malone J. (2020). X-rays for medical imaging: Radiation protection, governance and ethics over 125 years. *Physica Medica.* 2020;79:47–64. doi.org/10.1016/j.ejmp.2020.09.012

35. Samuel VJ, Gibikote S, Kirupakaran H. The routine pre-employment screening chest radiograph: Should it be routine? *The Indian Journal of Radiology & Imaging.* 2016 Jul;26(3):402. doi.org/10.4103/0971-3026.190409

36. Jasper A, Gibikote S, Kirupakaran H, Christopher DJ, Mathews P. Is routine pre-entry chest radiograph necessary in a high tuberculosis prevalence country?. *Journal of Postgraduate Medicine.* 2020 Apr;66(2):90.PMID:32270779

37. Thomas JP, Srinivasan A, Wickramarachchi CS, Dhesi PK, Hung YM, Kamath AV. Evaluating the national PPE guidance for NHS healthcare workers during the COVID-19 pandemic. *Clinical Medicine.* 2020 May;20(3):242. doi.org/10.7861/clinmed.2020-0143

38. McLeod M, Sandiford P, Kvizhinadze G, Bartholomew K, Crengle S. Impact of low-dose CT screening for lung cancer on ethnic health inequities in New Zealand: A cost-effectiveness analysis. *BMJ Open.* 2020 Sep 1;10(9):e037145. doi.org/10.1136/bmjopen-2020-037145

39. Piersiala K, Akst LM, Hillel AT, Best SR. ct Lung Screening in patients with laryngeal cancer. *Scientific Reports.* 2020 Mar 13;10(1):1–8. doi.org/10.1038/s41598-020-61511-3

40. Shen H. Low-dose CT for lung cancer screening: Opportunities and challenges. *Frontiers of Medicine.* 2018 Feb;12(1):116–21. doi.org/10.1007/s11684-017-0600-1

41. Rampinelli C, De Marco P, Origgi D, Maisonneuve P, Casiraghi M, Veronesi G, Spaggiari L, Bellomi M. Exposure to low dose computed tomography for lung cancer screening and risk of cancer: Secondary analysis of trial data and risk-benefit analysis. *BMJ.* 2017 Feb 8;356.

42. Abuelhia E. Awareness of ionizing radiation exposure among junior doctors and senior medical students in radiological investigations. *Journal of Radiological Protection.* 2016;37(1):59. http://iopscience.iop.org/0952-4746/37/1/59

43. Arora R, Arora AJ. Justification of whole-body CT in polytrauma patients, can clinical examination help selecting patients? *Quantitative Imaging in Medicine and Surgery.* 2019;9(4):636–41. doi.org/10.21037/qims.2019.04.02

44. Remedios D. Justification: How to get referring physicians involved. *Radiation Protection Dosimetry.* 2011 Sep 1;147(1–2):47–51.

45. Rehani MM, Yang K, Melick ER, Heil J, Šalát D, Sensakovic WF, Liu B. Patients undergoing recurrent CT scans: Assessing the magnitude. *European Radiology.* 2020 Apr;30(4):1828–36.

46. Autier P, Boniol M. Mammography screening: A major issue in medicine. *European Journal of Cancer.* 2018;90:34–62. doi.org/10.1016/j.ejca.2017.11.002

47. Hofmann B. (2020). Informing about mammographic screening: Ethical challenges and suggested solutions. *Bioethics*. 2020;34(5):483–92. doi.org/10.1111/bioe.12676

48. Seaman K, Dzidic PL, Castell E, Saunders C, Breen LJ. Subject positions in screening mammography and implications for informed choice. *Psychology & Health*. 2021 Apr 3;36(4):478–95. doi.org/10.1080/08870446.2020.1766043

49. Beckett KR, Moriarity AK, Langer JM. Safe use of contrast media: What the radiologist needs to know. *Radiographics*. 2015 Oct;35(6):1738–50. doi.org/10.1148/rg.2015150033

50. Speck U. *X-ray contrast media: Overview, use and pharmaceutical aspects.* Springer Nature; Cham, Switzerland, 2018.

51. De Simone B, Ansaloni L, Sartelli M, Gaiani F, Leandro G, De' Angelis GL, Di Mario F, Coccolini F, Catena F. Is the risk of contrast-induced nephropathy a real contraindication to perform intravenous contrast enhanced Computed Tomography for non-traumatic acute abdomen in Emergency Surgery Department? *Acta Biomedica*. 2018 Dec 17;89(9-S):158–72. doi.org/10.23750/abm.v89i9-S.7891. PMID:30561410

52. Cartocci G, Santurro A, La Russa R, Guglielmi G, Frati P, Fineschi V. The choice of gadolinium-based contrast agents: A radiologist's responsibility between pharmaceutical equivalence and bioethical issues. *Symmetry*. 2017 Nov;9(11):287. doi.org/10.3390/sym9110287

53. Costantino MT, Romanini L, Gaeta F, Stacul F, Valluzzi RL, Passamonti M, Bonadonna P, Cerri G, Pucci S, Ricci P, Savi E. SIRM-SIAAIC consensus, an Italian document on management of patients at risk of hypersensitivity reactions to contrast media. *Clinical and Molecular Allergy*. 2020 Dec;18(1):1–10. doi.org/10.1186/s12948-020-00128-3

54. Brady Z, Scoullar H, Grinsted B, Ewert K, Kavnoudias H, Jarema A, Crocker J, Wills R, Houston G, Law M, Varma D. Technique, radiation safety and image quality for chest X-ray imaging through glass and in mobile settings during the COVID-19 pandemic. *Physical and Engineering Sciences in Medicine*. 2020 Sep;43(3):765–79. doi.org/10.1007/s13246-020-00899-8

55. Mattijssen-Horstink L, Langeraar JJ, Mauritz GJ, van der Stappen W, Baggelaar M, Tan EC. Radiologic discrepancies in diagnosis of fractures in a Dutch teaching emergency department: A retrospective analysis. *Scandinavian Journal of Trauma, Resuscitation and Emergency Medicine*. 2020 Dec;28:1–7. doi.org/10.1186/s13049-020-00727-8

56. Opancina V, Vojinović, R. (2018). Medical error: General term and its overview in radiology. *Medicinskičasopis*. 2018;52(1):22–5. doi.org/10.5937/mckg52-16836

57. Waite S, Scott JM, Legasto A, Kolla S, Gale B, Krupinski EA. Systemic error in radiology. *American Journal of Roentgenology*. 2017;209(3):629–39. doi.org/10.2214/AJR.16.17719

58. Brown SD, Bruno MA, Shyu JY, Eisenberg R, Abujudeh H, Norbash A, Gallagher TH. Error disclosure and apology in radiology: The case for further dialogue. *Radiology*. 2019 Oct;293(1):30–5. doi.org/10.1148/radiol.2019190126

59. Brown C, Neep MJ, Pozzias E, McPhail SM. Reducing risk in the emergency department: A 12-month prospective longitudinal study of radiographer preliminary image evaluations. *Journal of Medical Radiation Sciences*. 2019 Sep;66(3):154–62. doi.org/10.1002/jmrs.341

60. Squibb K, Smith A, Dalton L, Bull RM. The 'radiographer–referrer game': Image interpretation dynamics in rural practice. *Journal of Medical Radiation Sciences*. 2016;63(1):17–22. doi.org/10.1002/jmrs.152

61. Murphy A, Liszewski B. Artificial intelligence and the medical radiation profession: How our advocacy must inform future practice. *Journal of Medical Imaging and Radiation Sciences*. 2019;50(4 Supplement 2):S15–9. doi.org/10.1016/j.jmir.2019.09.001

62. Australian Radiation Protection and Nuclear Safety Agency (2002) *Radiation protection series, 1. Recommendations for limiting exposure to ionizing radiation (1995), guidance note NOHSC:3022(1995). National standard for limiting occupational exposure to ionizing radiation, NOHSC:1013(1995).* National Occupational Health and Safety Commission. ARPANSA, Yallambie, Victoria.

63. Mathur S, Pillenahalli Maheshwarappa R, Fouladirad S, Metwally O, Mukherjee P, Lin AW, ... Ditkofsky NG. Emergency imaging in pregnancy and lactation. *Canadian Association of Radiologists Journal*. 2020;71(3):396–402. doi.org/10.1177/0846537120906482

64. Tomà P, Bartoloni A, Salerno S, Granata C, Cannatà V, Magistrelli A, Arthurs OJ. Protecting sensitive patient groups from imaging using ionizing radiation: Effects during pregnancy, in fetal life and childhood. *La radiologia medica*. 2014;124:736–44. doi.org/10.1007/s11547-019-01034-8

65. Paolicchi F, Miniati F, Bastian, L, Faggioni L, Ciaramella A, Creonti I, Sottocornola C, Dionisi C, Caramella D. Assessment of radiation protection awareness and knowledge about radiological examination doses among Italian radiographers. *Insights Imaging*. 2016;7:233–42. doi.org/10.1007/s13244-015-0445-6

66. Ciraj-Bjelac O, Carinou E, Ferrari P, Gingaume M, Merce MS, O'Connor U. Occupational exposure of the eye lens in interventional procedures: How to assess and manage radiation dose. *Journal of the American College of Radiology*. 2016 Nov 1;13(11):1347–53. doi.org/10.1016/j.jacr.2016.06.015

67. Group, SFR-IA, French Radiology Community. Artificial intelligence and medical imaging 2018: French Radiology Community white paper. *Diagnostic and Interventional Imaging*. 2018 Nov 1;99(11):727–42. doi.org/10.1016/j.diii.2018.10.003

68. Portelli JL, McNulty, JP, Bezzina P, Rainford L. Benefit-risk communication in paediatric imaging: What do referring physicians, radiographers and radiologists think, say and do? *Radiography*. 2018;24(1):33–40. doi.org/10.1016/j.radi.2017.08.009

69. Challen R, Low LF, McEntee MF. Dementia patient care in the diagnostic medical imaging department. *Radiography*. 2018 Oct 1;24(Supplement 1):S33–42. doi.org/10.1016/j.radi.2018.05.012

70. Fisher CB. A relational perspective on ethics-in-science decision making for research with vulnerable populations. *IRB: Ethics & Human Research*. 1997 Sep 1;19(5):1–4. doi.org/10.2307/3564120

71. Caillé JM. La radiologiepeut-ellesurvivre? Doit-ellesurvivre? La chronique d une mort annoncée. *Journal of Radiology*. 1999;80:1523–5.

72. Moores BM, Regulla D. A review of the scientific basis for radiation protection of the patient. *Radiation Protection Dosimetry*. 2011 Sep 1;147(1–2):22–9. doi.org/10.1093/rpd/ncr262

73. Doudenkova V, Pipon JC. Duty to inform and informed consent in diagnostic radiology: How ethics and law can better guide practice. In *Hec forum*; 2016 Mar 1; 28(1):75–94. Springer Netherlands. doi.org/10.1007/s10730-015-9275-7

74. Høilund-Carlsen PF. The good rays: Let them shine! *European Journal of Nuclear Medicine and Molecular Imaging*. 2019;46:271–5. doi.org/10.1007/s00259-018-4233-7

75. Protection R. ICRP publication 103. *Ann ICRP*. 2007;37(2.4):2. http://www.elsevier. com/wps/find/bookdescription.cws_home/713998/description#description

76. Goguen J. (2016). Health literacy and patient preparation in radiology. *Journal of Medical Imaging and Radiation Sciences*. 2016;47(3):283–6. doi.org/10.1016/j.jmir. 2016.06.002

77. Ukkola L., Kyngäs H., Henner A., Oikarinen H. (2020). Barriers to not informing patients about radiation in connection with radiological examinations: Radiographers' opinion. *Radiography*. 2020;26(2):e114–9. doi.org/10.1016/j.radi.2019.12.005

78. Abuelhia E, Alghamdi A. Evaluation of arising exposure of ionizing radiation from computed tomography and the associated health concerns. *Journal of Radiation Research and Applied Sciences*. 2020 Jan 1;13(1):295–300. doi.org/10.1080/16878507. 2020.1728962

79. Chew C, Cannon P, O'Dwyer PJ. Radiology for medical students (1925–2018): An overview. *BJR|Open*. 2020 Feb;2(1):20190050. doi.org/10.1259/bjro.20190050

80. Matheny ME, Whicher D, Israni ST. Artificial intelligence in health care: A report from the National Academy of Medicine. *JAMA*. 2020 Feb 11;323(6):509–10. doi.org/10.10 01/jama.2019.21579

81. Woznitza N. Artificial intelligence and the radiographer/radiological technologist profession: A joint statement of the international society of radiographers and radiological technologists and the European federation of radiographer societies. *Radiography*. 2020 May 1;26(2):93–5.

82. Recht MP, Dewey M, Dreyer K, Langlot, C, Niessen W, Prainsack B, Smith JJ. (2020). Integrating artificial intelligence into the clinical practice of radiology: Challenges and recommendations. *European Radiology*. 2020;1–9. doi.org/10.1007/s00330-020-06672-5

83. Allen Jr B, Seltzer SE, Langlotz, CP, Dreyer, KP, Summers, RM, Petrick, N., ... Kandarpa K. (2019). A road map for translational research on artificial intelligence in medical imaging: From the 2018 National Institutes of Health/RSNA/ACR/The Academy Workshop. *Journal of the American College of Radiology*. 2019;16(9):1179–89. doi. org/10.1016/j.jacr.2019.04.014

84. Carlton RR, Adler AM. *Principles of radiographic imaging (book only)*. Cengage Learning; 2012 Jan 13.

2

Medical Imaging and Computer-Aided Diagnosis

Megha P. Arakeri, Lakshmana, and Sunil Kumar Manvi

Introduction

Medical imaging plays an important role in healthcare as it can help the physician to examine the internal details of the human body in a non-invasive manner. It provides useful information on patients' medical conditions and helps to investigate causes of their symptoms and diseases.[1] Various imaging modalities like CT, MRI, and ultrasound are widely used in hospitals, clinics, and diagnostic centres to acquire the image of the internal organs. Analysis of these images is a crucial task because these images are taken at low energy and also may be affected by noise. If these images are taken at a high energy, then it may harm the patient. Further, daily, large numbers of images are generated in hospitals, and hence analysis of these images by the radiologist is tedious. Effective interpretation of these images requires an experienced doctor. Due to these subjective factors and the poor quality of images, visual analysis of these images by a radiologist may lead to inaccurate results. In order to overcome these drawbacks, there is a strong demand for computer-aided diagnosis (CAD) systems in hospitals.

In order to attain a more reliable and accurate diagnosis, various computer-aided diagnosis systems have been developed to assist radiologists in the interpretation of medical images. The basic concept of CAD is to process the medical image automatically and provide a computer output as a second opinion to assist radiologists' image interpretation.[2] Currently, researchers are focusing on the design and development of medical imaging and analysis systems by using digital image processing tools and the techniques of artificial intelligence, which can detect abnormal features, classify them, and provide visual proofs to the radiologists.[3] Thus, CAD can be used to assist the radiologist in detection, diagnosis, and surgical planning. A lot of research is going on in developing CAD for examining the

DOI: 10.1201/9781003112068-2

brain, liver, kidney, colon, bone, etc. CAD systems for the detection of breast lesions on mammograms have been developed and are commercially available. These systems have received FDA approval for clinical use.[4]

The rest of the chapter is organized as follows. The section "Medical Imaging Techniques" discusses the working principles of medical imaging techniques. The section "Computer-Aided Design" presents details of computer-aided diagnosis systems. Various clinical applications are discussed in the section "Clinical Applications". Finally, challenges and future directions are discussed in the following section.

Medical Imaging Techniques

Once a disease is clinically suspected based on symptoms, radiologic evaluation is required to determine the location, type, and extent of the disease and its relationship to the surrounding structures. This information is very important in deciding on the treatment option. It also helps in monitoring treatment response as well as the patient's prognosis. Medical imaging has played a major role in clinical diagnosis and treatment for years, allowing radiologists to examine specific sections of the human body without resorting to invasive surgical procedures. Images may be enhanced by introducing contrast agents during image acquisition to provide clear information about the abnormal region on the organ being scanned. The working principles, benefits, and drawbacks of some widely used important imaging methods are given below.

Ultrasonography

Ultrasonography is used for imaging soft tissues, and its working principle is based on high-frequency sound waves called ultrasound whose frequency lies above the audible range of normal human hearing, about 20 kHz. The frequency used in diagnostic ultrasound is typically in the range of 2 to 18 MHz.[5] In order to acquire the image of the organ, a transducer sends a small pulse of ultrasound into the body. As the ultrasound waves penetrate tissues of different acoustic impedances along the path of transmission, some are reflected back to the transducer (echo signals) and some continue to penetrate deeper. The echo signals returned from many sequential coplanar pulses are processed and combined to generate an image. The advantages of ultrasonography are good soft tissue contrast, availability, relatively low cost, and absence of ionizing radiation. It also provides real-time scanning of soft tissue structures. The limitations of ultrasonography are operator dependency and poor spatial resolution of the image due to blurring.

Computed Tomography

The CT imaging technique can be used to detect tumours, and its working principle is based on passing multiple X-ray beams at different angles through the body to build up a cross-sectional image of the organ.[6] The CT imaging system is comprised of a motorized table that moves the patient through a circular opening and an X-ray machine that rotates around the patient as he moves through. Detectors record the radiation exiting the patient's body, and this creates an X-ray snapshot. Many different snapshots are collected during one complete rotation of the X-ray machine, and then the computer assembles the series of X-ray images into a cross section. Thus, a CT scan produces a series of cross-sectional images of the organ being scanned. In conventional CT, the X-ray tube rotates around the patient while the table is immobile. After one scan is over, the table moves, and the procedure is repeated; thus it requires more image acquisition time. Recent technological advances in CT technology, such as spiral and multi-detector CT, have further improved the performance of conventional CT scanners in terms of image acquisition speed and resolution.[7] In spiral CT, X-ray tube rotation and patient table translation are performed simultaneously. Multi-detector CT uses multiple detector rows as opposed to one detector row in spiral CT, and thus it can obtain multiple slices in a single rotation.

The advantages of CT are fast image acquisition, the imaging of soft tissues as well as bones, and lower cost. The main limitation is that it uses ionizing radiation to generate images of the organ and hence cannot be used for scanning pregnant women. Also, sometimes the contrast agents used during CT imaging lead to allergic reactions in patients.

Magnetic Resonance Imaging

The MRI technique can be used to acquire a set of cross-sectional images of the brain as well as liver. It makes use of magnetic fields and radio waves to acquire the image of the organ being scanned.[8] The MRI unit consists of a large cylindrical shaped tube surrounded by a circular magnet. An electric current passes through the coils of the unit to create a magnetic field. In order to perform the MRI scan, the patient is made to lie within the electromagnetic field created. The human body is mainly composed of water containing hydrogen atoms. Normally, the nuclei of the body's atoms spin on axes aligned in different directions. But the MRI's powerful magnetic field realigns the protons of the body's hydrogen atoms so that they all spin along the same axis. The MRI machine sends radio waves into the area of the body being scanned and causes the atoms to change from low energy to high energy states. When the radio waves are switched off, the atoms fall back to their low energy states. As they do this, they lose their energy, giving off signals which are then picked up by the MRI machine. A computer processes these signals and produces an image of the organ being scanned.

MRI uses many different types of images, such as T1-weighted, T2-weighted, diffusion-weighted, and magnetic susceptibility-weighted. These images are produced with different types of imaging parameters, such as repetition time (TR) and echo time (TE). T1-weighted and T2-weighted are the most commonly used MRI images for diagnosing brain/liver tumours.[9] On a T1-weighted image, water appears dark and fat appears bright, whereas on a T2-weighted image, water appears bright and fat appears dark. The advantages of MRI are the absence of ionizing radiations, high resolution, and soft tissue contrast. The contrast material used in MRI exams is less likely to produce an allergic reaction. The disadvantages of MRI are the long examination time, relatively high cost, and limited availability. MRI is rarely used as the first diagnostic modality, except for brain and soft tissue tumours. Indications for MRI are usually difficult clinical cases that are not resolved after US or CT examinations.

Nuclear Imaging

Nuclear imaging uses low doses of radioactive substances to detect abnormalities. During nuclear imaging, the radioactive tracer, which is formulated to accumulate in specific organs, bones, or tissues, is injected into the body.[10] Sensors in the scanner detect the radioactivity as the tracer accumulates in different regions of the organ. A computer uses the data gathered by the sensors to construct multi-coloured images that show where the compound acts in the organ. Allergies, side effects, and other reactions are extremely rare in nuclear imaging, as very small doses of tracer are used.

Two major instruments used in nuclear imaging for the detection of cancer are PET and SPECT scanners. PET and SPECT rely on similar principles to produce images of the organ. The important differences in instrumentation, radiochemistry, and experimental applications are dictated by differences in their respective physics of photon emission. Generally, SPECT tracers deteriorate more slowly than PET tracers. Hence, SPECT requires longer scan periods than PET. The PET is more versatile than SPECT and produces more detailed images with a higher degree of resolution.

Computer-Aided Diagnosis (CAD)

CAD is an interdisciplinary field which combines medical imaging with image processing, pattern recognition, computer science, and artificial intelligence technologies.[11] CAD can be defined as a diagnosis made by a radiologist who uses the output from a computerized analysis of medical images as a second opinion in detecting disease and making diagnostic decisions. Thus, CAD is often classified into two major groups: computer-aided detection (CADe) and computer-aided diagnosis (CADx). CADe focuses on detection/localization of disease on medical images, and CADx focuses on identifying the type of disease.[12] The radiologist's image interpreting sensitivity can be increased and accurate diagnosis can be made with the support of a CAD system. Hence, deadly diseases like cancer can be detected in early stages and cured without much difficulty with the help of a CAD system.

As shown in Figure 2.1, computer-aided diagnosis based on medical images consists of the following steps: image acquisition, pre-processing, segmentation, feature extraction and selection, and classification. The medical images acquired through imaging techniques, such as US, CT, MRI, PET, or SPECT, are input to the CAD system for diagnosis of the disease. The steps of CAD are explained as follows.

Pre-Processing

Images acquired by medical imaging devices may contain noise, and this makes the image analysis very difficult. Thus, the pre-processing step makes the image suitable for further processing by improving the quality of the image. It involves various tasks such as deblurring, noise reduction, and contrast enhancement.

Segmentation

In order to characterize the disease, the location of the abnormality on the given medical image has to be identified. Thus, the segmentation step subdivides the image into different regions based on certain properties to delineate the region of interest in the given image.

Feature Extraction and Selection

In this step, various features of the segmented region are extracted to represent the characteristics of the disease. The features extracted may be shape, size, texture, average

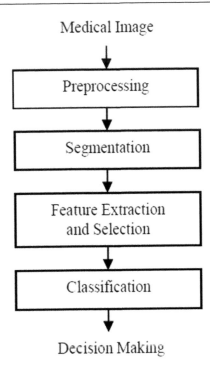

Medical Image

Preprocessing

Segmentation

Feature Extraction and Selection

Classification

Decision Making

Figure 2.1 The computer-aided diagnosis process.

grey level, etc. However, a large number of features degrade the performance of the classifier. Thus, the feature selection step is required to reduce the dimensionality of the feature space and keep only a set of features which are most discriminating and helpful for the classifier in identifying the type of disease.

Classification

The selected features of the segmented region are fed to the classifier to determine the class of the disease, and the classifier used can be supervised or unsupervised. A supervised classifier identifies the type of the disease based on the given examples, whereas an unsupervised classifier does not need any examples or training to identify the type of disease. Finally, the radiologist makes the diagnostic decision on the suspicious region in the medical image based upon the output of the CAD system.

Clinical Applications

Clinical acceptance of the CAD system depends on its accuracy. Thus, in order to make the CAD system more effective and helpful, researchers are trying to integrate advanced technologies like cognitive computing, deep learning, artificial intelligence, etc. CAD systems used in healthcare are meant to give a second opinion for the clinician in disease diagnosis. It must be automatic without any manual intervention, giving real-time diagnosis and 100% diagnostic accuracy. Currently, CAD systems are used in the diagnosis of breast cancer, congenital heart disease, Alzheimer's disease, brain tumours, pulmonary nodules, diabetic retinopathy, etc. Some of the systems or methods developed by researchers are discussed below.

Breast Cancer

Worldwide breast cancer is the second leading cause of death among women.[13] Early detection of breast cancer may improve the survival rate of the patient. Mammography uses low-dose X-ray during breast examination and is used as a screening tool for breast cancer diagnosis in the early stage. But mammography has a low detection rate, and its results depend on the patient's age and breast density.[14] Hence, visual analysis of these mammogram images by a radiologist may increase false positive rates and may lead to unnecessary biopsy. In order to overcome this problem many CAD systems have been developed to automatically analyse these medical images in an effective manner.[15–17] Recently, contrast-enhanced digital mammograms have emerged as a promising imaging modality in breast cancer imaging. They use iodinated contrast materials for the visualization of breast neovascularity. The technique provides high spatial resolution and information on physiological function with the best operation speed and low cost.[18]

Congenital Heart Disease

Congenital heart disease (CHD) refers to the structural and functional abnormalities of the heart at birth. Early detection of CHD is very important since it is one of the major causes of foetal death. Without timely diagnosis and treatment, children with CHD would die within a year after birth. Therefore, accurate and early detection of CHD is crucial.[19] Early detection of CHD allows appropriate clinical interventions to be made either during pregnancy or in planning the appropriate delivery time and mode. Undetected cases result in the birth of a baby with heart defects or result in serious complications within a few years of birth. CT, MRI, and ultrasound are the imaging techniques used for the detection and analysis of CHD.[20] There is a great focus on utilizing non-invasive and non-radiation techniques for the detection of heart diseases. Among these imaging techniques, ultrasound is the best method for imaging the foetal heart as it is radiation free, non-invasive, and low cost. Hence, ultrasound imaging modality is commonly used for monitoring the growth of the foetus and detecting any abnormalities. However, manual interpretation of these images is a challenging task since these images are affected by speckle noise. Hence, detecting any heart abnormalities depends mainly on the expertise of the radiologist. This has grabbed a great deal of attention from researchers on developing computer-aided diagnostic systems/ automated methods to assist clinicians in the diagnosis of CHD and minimizing the chances of false predictions.[21-23]

Alzheimer's Disease

Alzheimer's disease (AD) is a progressively neuro-degenerative disorder, and it is the main cause of dementia in elderly people worldwide. It is expected to increase drastically in the coming years due to the growth of the older population.[24] It gradually deteriorates the cognitive and behavioural capacities of the patient. Currently, there is no clinical method that can predict whether a particular person will develop the disease. With the advent of several effective treatments of AD symptoms, the current situation has emphasized the need for early recognition. Imaging modalities such as MRI, PET, and SPECT are very effective in the detection of AD.[25] A CAD system can help to perform an early diagnosis which is crucial for mitigating the effects of AD. Several diagnostic tools and approaches have been developed in order to detect early changes, clarify the underlying mechanisms, and inform neuro-protective interventions aimed at slowing down the extent of the disease.[26–28] Several computational intelligence techniques, data fusion, and multimodal approaches are used to improve the accuracy of these automated methods.

Challenges and Future Directions

The challenges that must be addressed for the development of an effective and efficient CAD system are as follows.

Disease Detection

The detection of an abnormal/affected region on a given medical image is challenging as the medical image shows other tissues or organs adjacent to the affected region. Some of the organs are very closely located and have similar intensities in medical images. In such cases it becomes difficult to segment the affected region, since the organ has to be detected and then its affected region. Hence, to properly delineate the diseased region on the medical image one should have knowledge about the characteristics of a medical image, the anatomy of the organ, and the difference between normal and abnormal tissues.

Automation

Since the aim of the CAD system is to provide computer assisted characterization of tissues, all phases in the CAD system from pre-processing to classification should be automatic. However, achieving this goal is difficult, since some phases like segmentation require input from the radiologist. Automating the segmentation task is challenging due to the complex anatomy and the diverse shapes of organs.

Accuracy

The important characteristic expected in the CAD system is to achieve high sensitivity in disease diagnosis with the fewest number of false positives. If the information given by the CAD system is flawed, then the radiologist's decision that is based on such information has the potential to be flawed as well. Thus, a large number of false positives would reduce the efficiency of the radiologist and clinical acceptance of the CAD system. But, to make the system more accurate, it needs to be trained with various types of cases, which is a difficult process.

Efficiency

In addition to accuracy, efficiency is also an important feature of the CAD system. In a clinical environment, routinely a large number of images are generated and thus the analysis of these images should be fast. If the CAD system is slower than the manual interpretation of images, then the radiologist does not find it useful. Early diagnosis of deadly diseases like cancer helps in providing the appropriate treatment at the right time and hence improves the survival chances of the patient.

Noisy Images

Images acquired from medical imaging modalities are usually affected by noise. The presence of noise corrupts the information in the image and thus increases the false positive rate in diagnosis. Hence, the CAD system must have denoising algorithms which eliminate the noise as well as retain the border and shape of regions in the medical image.

Learning from Radiologists

A radiologist uses multiple criteria for diagnosing a suspected region on medical images. Although algorithms could be developed by learning from training examples, algorithms are likely to be more successful if based on features that are proven clinically relevant. The features which radiologists find useful include anatomic knowledge, image characteristics, shape, and texture. Hence, incorporating the knowledge of the radiologist into the CAD system is a challenging task. After extensive review of the existing CAD systems, the following are the research issues identified for developing an automatic, effective, and efficient CAD system for assisting the radiologist in clinical decision making.

The accuracy of disease-affected region segmentation determines the eventual success or failure of computerized medical image analysis tasks like diagnosis, volume analysis, and surgical planning. Most of the existing segmentation methods are manual or semi-automatic. These methods are time consuming and do not automate the entire diagnosis process of the CAD system, since they require manual intervention in the segmentation. But hospitals are in need of fully automatic diagnosis systems with better accuracy compared to the analysis of the disease by the physician. Though some automatic segmentation techniques exist, they do not provide the accuracy required in the medical domain. Hence, there is a need to develop a fully automatic, accurate, and efficient segmentation method for the detection of diseases/affected regions on medical images.

In an effort to deliver more effective treatment, clinicians are continuously seeking greater accuracy in the pathological characterization of abnormal region tissues from imaging investigations. Hence, to build an effective CAD system for correctly classifying diseases, it is necessary to present all the features of the affected region to the CAD system. The existing methods employ few features for characterizing the pathology of the region, and no method uses all the features in a comprehensive manner. However, the use of all the heterogeneous information leads to high-dimensional feature vectors and in turn degrades the diagnostic accuracy of CAD systems significantly. Therefore, a reliable feature selection technique is needed for providing compact and discriminating descriptors. Another observation is that the majority of the existing techniques analyse the performance of different classifiers separately and under some specific contexts. However, a decision support system based on an ensemble classifier would be more effective compared to individual classifiers alone. Now, the research focus is on investigating the effectiveness of the features extracted from heterogeneous imaging modalities (such as MRI, CT, and ultrasonography) in the development of CAD. More extensive training using larger datasets is expected to further improve the disease characterization ability of CAD systems.

Conclusion

This chapter presented the concepts of different medical imaging techniques and CAD systems. Currently, medical imaging techniques are advancing to provide better quality images for effective diagnosis. Many CAD systems have been approved by the FDA for use in lung CT, virtual colonoscopy, and breast MRI. CAD is also undergoing transition from a pure detection device to a diagnostic one with the advancement of technologies like artificial intelligence and cognitive computing. Effective CAD systems along with advanced medical imaging techniques provide an automated diagnostic tool for assisting the radiologist in accurate clinical decision making. This also helps clinicians in detecting deadly diseases in early stages and thus improves the survival rate of patients.

References

1. Laal M. Innovation process in medical imaging. *Procedia - Social and Behavioral Sciences*. 2013 June;81:60–4.

2. Suzuki K. A review of computer-aided diagnosis in thoracic and colonic imaging. *Quantitative Imaging in Medicine and Surgery*. 2012 Sep;2(3):163–76.

3. Gao Y, Geras KJ, Lewin AA, Moy L. New frontiers: An update on computer-aided diagnosis for breast imaging in the age of artificial intelligence. *AJR - American Roentgen Ray Society*. 2019 Feb;212(2):300–7.

4. Retson TA, Eghtedari M. Computer-aided detection/diagnosis in breast imaging: A focus on the evolving FDA regulations for using software as a medical device. *Current Radiology Reports*. 2020 May;8(6):1–7.

5. Gitto S, Grassi G, De Angelis C, Monaco CG, Sdao S, Sardanelli F, Sconfienza LM, Mauri G. A computer-aided diagnosis system for the assessment and characterization of low-to-high suspicion thyroid nodules on ultrasound. *La radiologia medica*. 2019 Feb;124(2):118–25.

6. Schmidt CW. CT scans: Balancing health risks and medical benefits. *Environmental Health Perspectives*. 2012 Mar;120(3):A118–21.

7. Ginat DT, Gupta R. Advances in computed tomography imaging technology. *Annual Review of Biomedical Engineering*. 2014 Jul;16:431–53.

8. Villanueva-Meyer JE, Mabray MC, Cha S. Current clinical brain tumor imaging. *Neurosurgery*. 2017 Sep;81(3):397–415.

9. Xiao Y, Paudel R, Liu J, Ma C, Zhang Z, Zhou S. MRI contrast agents: Classification and application (Review). *International Journal of Molecular Medicine*. 2016 Sep;38(5):1319–26.

10. Zanzonico P. Principles of nuclear medicine imaging: Planar, SPECT, PET, multi-modality, and autoradiography systems. *Radiation Research*. 2012 Apr;177(4):349–64.

11. Santos MK, Ferreira Júnior JR, Wada DT, Tenório APM, Barbosa MHN, Marques PMA. Artificial intelligence, machine learning, computer-aided diagnosis, and radiomics: Advances in imaging towards to precision medicine. *Radiologia Brasileira.* 2019 Nov–Dec;52(6):387–96.

12. Firmino M, Angelo G, Morais H, Dantas MR, Valentim R. Computer-aided detection (CADe) and diagnosis (CADx) system for lung cancer with likelihood of malignancy. *Biomedical Engineering Online.* 2016 Jan;15(1):1–7.

13. American Cancer Society. *Breast cancer facts and figures 2019–2020 [Internet].* American Cancer Society, Atlanta; 2019. Available from: https://www.cancer.org/research/cancer-facts-statistics.html

14. Longo R, Tonutti M, Rigon L, Arfelli F, Dreossi D, Quai E, Zanconati F, Castelli E, Tromba G, Cova MA. Clinical study in phase- contrast mammography: Image-quality analysis. *Philosophical Transactions of the Royal Society A: Mathematical, Physical and Engineering Sciences.* 2014 Jan;372(2010):20130025.

15. Rizzi M, D'Aloia M, Castagnolo B. Health care CAD systems for breast microcalcification cluster detection. *Journal of Medical and Biological Engineering.* 2012 Jun;32(3):147–56.

16. Ohuchi N, Suzuki A, Sobue T, Kawai M, Yamamoto S, Zheng YF, et al. Sensitivity and specificity of mammography and adjunctive ultrasonography to screen for breast cancer in the Japan Strategic Anti-cancer Randomized Trial (J-START): A randomised controlled trial. *Lancet.* 2016 Jan;387(10016):341–8.

17. Watanabe AT, Lim V, Vu HX, Chim R, Weise E, Liu J, Bradley WG, Comstock CE. Improved cancer detection using artificial intelligence: A retrospective evaluation of missed cancers on mammography. *Journal Digit Imaging.* 2019 Aug;32(4):625–37.

18. Ghaderi KF, Phillips J, Perry H, Lotf P, Mehta TS. Contrast-enhanced mammography: Current applications and future directions. *RadioGraphics.* 2019 Nov;39(7):1907–20.

19. JingjingLv, DB, Lei H, Shi G, Wang H, Zhu F, Wen C, Zhang Q, Fu L, Gu X, Yuan J. Artificial intelligence-assisted auscultation in detecting congenital heart disease. *European Heart Journal - Digital Health.* 2021 Mar;2(1):119–24.

20. Sachdeva S, Gupta SK. Imaging modalities in congenital heart disease. *Indian Journal of Pediatrics.* 2020 May;87(5):385–97.

21. Sundaresan V, Bridge C, Ioannou C, Noble J. Automated characterization of the fetal heart in ultrasound images using fully convolutional neural networks. In *IEEE 14th International Symposium on Biomedical Imaging;* 2017 Apr 18–21; 2017, IEEE, Melbourne, VIC, Australia (pp. 671–4).

22. Sridar P, Kumar A, Quinton A, Nanan R, Kim J, Krishnakumar R. Decision fusion-based fetal ultrasound image plane classification using convolutional neural networks. *Ultrasound in Medicine and Biology.* 2019 May;45(5):1259–73.

23. Dozen A, Komatsu M, Sakai A, Komatsu R, Shozu K, Machino H, Yasutomi S, Arakaki T, Asada K, Kaneko S, Matsuoka R. Image segmentation of the ventricular septum in fetal cardiac ultrasound videos based on deep learning using time-series information. *Biomolecules.* 2020 Nov;10(11):1526.

24. Ramírez J, Chaves R, Gorriz JM, Lopez M, Lvarez IÁ, Salas-Gonzalez D, Segovia F, Padilla P. Computer aided diagnosis of the Alzheimer's disease combining SPECT-based feature selection and random forest classifiers. In *IEEE Nuclear Science Symposium Conference Record (NSS/MIC)*, 2009 Nov 1-Oct 24; 2009, IEEE, Orlando, FL, USA (pp. 2738–42).

25. Padilla P, López M, Górriz J, Ramírez J, Salas-González D, Álvarez I. The Alzheimer's disease neuroimaging initiative. NMF-SVM based CAD tool applied to functional brain images for the diagnosis of Alzheimer's disease. *IEEE Transactions on Medical Imaging*. 2012 Feb;31(2):207–16.

26. Dessouky MM, Elrashidy MA, Taha TE, Abdelkader HM. Computer-aided diagnosis system for Alzheimer's disease using different discrete transform techniques. *American Journal of Alzheimer's Disease & Other Dementias®*. 2016 May;31(3):282–93.

27. Karami V, Nittari G, Amenta F. Neuroimaging computer-aided diagnosis systems for Alzheimer's disease. *International Journal of Imaging Systems and Technology*. 2019 Mar;29(1):83–94.

28. Lazli L, Boukadoum M, Mohamed OA. A survey on computer-aided diagnosis of brain disorders through MRI based on machine learning and data mining methodologies with an emphasis on alzheimer disease diagnosis and the contribution of the multimodal fusion. *Applied Sciences*. 2020 Mar;10(5):1894.

3

X- and Gamma Ray Imaging (CT, PET and SPEC, Scintigraphy, and Radiography)
Benefits and Risks

Octavian G. Duliu

Introduction

The problem of evidencing the internal structure of optically opaque objects was of maximum importance, especially with the development of the Industrial Revolution and the advent of modern medicine. But, until the discovery of radioactivity and X-ray, both at the end of the 19th century, this problem seemed unsolvable.

Indeed, with the discovery of X-ray by Wilhelm Konrad Röntgen in 1895 [1] and of gamma rays in 1900 by Paul Villard [2], it was possible to reveal with enough clarity the internal forms of the human body (Figure 3.1). This was due to the fact that both X- and gamma rays are the same type of electromagnetic radiation whose energy is many orders of magnitude higher than the binding energy of atoms in molecules. This makes this kind of electromagnetic radiation extremely penetrating and capable of passing through objects whose thicknesses are of the order of several decimetres, i.e., the size of the human body.

With respect to other nuclear radiation such as alpha or beta rays, X- and gamma rays are quanta of electromagnetic and therefore, have a specific mode of interaction by singular acts, when the incident particle can transfer partially or totally their energy, both X- and gamma rays presenting an exponential type attenuation when passed through objects. As a result

DOI: 10.1201/9781003112068-3

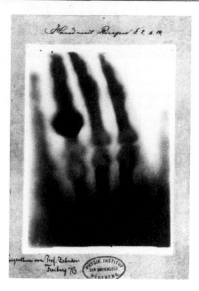

Figure 3.1 The first radiography—Hand mit Ringen (Hand with Rings): the radiography of the left hand of Anna Bertha Ludwig, the W.K. Röntgen's wife, as presented to Professor Ludwig Zehnder of the Physik Institut, University of Freiburg, on 1 January 1896 (https://en.wikipedia.org/wiki/File:First_medical_X-ray_by_Wilhelm_R%C3%B6ntgen_of_his_wife_Anna_Bertha_Ludwig%27s_hand_-_18951222.gif).

of this peculiarity, always a certain fraction of the incident radiation will cross the object, carrying in this way the information on its internal structure. Therefore, the object acts as a modulator of the incident radiation, of which spatial distribution on a section normal to the incident beam will reflect the internal nonuniformity of the investigated body. By using an appropriate image detector for the transmitted radiation such as a radiographic film or a solid-state detector like an image plate or flat panel detector, the emerging radiation is converted into a radiographic image.

In forming the radiographic image, the decisive role is played by the mode in which high-energy electromagnetic energy interacts with the investigated object. For energies commonly used in human examination, i.e., between 20 and 150 keV, the X- and gamma ray photons interact by three different mechanisms whose contribution to the total interaction depends on the radiation energy as well as on the object density and average atomic number [3]. These peculiarities permitted evidencing, in a distinct mode, the shape and structure of different constituents of the investigated body.

The radiographic examination can be done in a transmissive geometry as classic radiography and computed tomography (CT) (Figure 3.2a,b) [4] or in an emissive one as in the case of scintigraphy [4], positron emission tomography (PET) [4], or single photon emission tomography (SPET) (Figure 3.2c,d) [4]. In the first case the investigated body is placed between the radiation source and detectors while in the second case, the radiation source is localized within the body itself in front of an appropriate radiation detector (Figure 3.2). In both cases the final product is a projection of the investigated body as in the case of radiography or stratigraphy or a set of projections which, further processed, generates a tomographic image. For this reason, all these methods can be characterized as projective ones.

In the case of radiography and its emissive equivalent—the scintigraphy—the final image representing the object projection onto the detector plane appears flat, devoid of any information concerning the spatial distribution of the object structure.

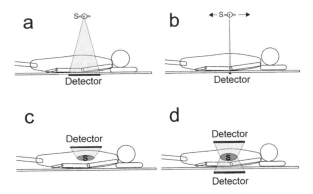

Figure 3.2 The transmissive (a,b) as well as the emissive (c,d) geometry in radiographic imaging. In the transmissive geometry, the body is placed between the source of radiation S and the detector, while the exposure can be done by a cone beam (a) when the detector can be a radiographic film or an image plate in the case of digital radiography or in a fan beam (b) when the detector consists of a diode array. In contrast, in the emissive geometry, the radiation source is located within the body as a distribution of a radiopharmaceutical while the detectors are outside the body single as in the case of planar scintigraphy or SPEC or by forming an opposite pair as in the case of PET.

This disadvantage was overcome by reconstructive imaging techniques such as CT, PET, and SPEC which, by using a series of object projections taken from different positions around the object, were able to reconstruct, using diverse algorithms, the spatial distribution of internal details of the investigated body initially in a section and later an entire volume.

It is worth mentioning that, while radiography and scintigraphy give direct images as they are produced by detectors, CT, PET, and SPEC reconstruct images from multiple projections which implies the use of various reconstruction algorithms, i.e., solving the inverse problem [5].

In spite of a greater breakthrough brought by X- and gamma ray imaging techniques in medical diagnosis, the use of high-energy ionizing radiation has some drawbacks which should be carefully taken into account when such an investigation is prescribed. These are intimately related with the amount of energy which the incident radiation transfers to the examined body. To generate radiographic images with an optimal contrast, the ratio of emergent radiation to incident should vary between 0.02 and 0.6, which means that between 40% and 98% of the energy of incident radiation will remain in the examined body. Here, the ionizing radiation can trigger a multitude of irreversible processes which could irremediably affect living cells, and especially DNA molecules.

For this reason, there is always a trade-off between the gain brought by a correct and rapid diagnosis and the detriment produced by irradiation, better postulated by the as low as reasonably achievable (ALARA) principle of radioprotection [6].

All these aspects will be further presented and discussed.

Interaction of X- and Gamma Rays with Matter

As mentioned before, X- and gamma rays represent the same kind of ultra-high-energy electromagnetic radiation which differ by the mechanism of their generation. X-rays are generated by braking high-energy electrons in the vicinity of target nuclei which is where its initial name of Bremsstrahlung comes from, while gamma rays are emitted by the daughter nuclei following a radioactive decay during a deexcitation process. At the same time, X-rays are emitted also when electrons from outer shells fill a vacancy in the inner shell of an atom. This kind of X-ray is called characteristic as their energy spectrum is specific for each element [7].

The difference between the production mechanisms of X- and gamma rays is reflected in their energy spectrum. While gamma rays have a discrete energy spectrum, the X-ray energy spectrum has a continuous component specific to brake radiation over which the peaks of characteristic radiation are superposed (Figure 3.3a). These differences are reflected by how they are produced and utilized in practice. X-rays are generated by X-ray generators or Coolidge tubes when a beam of accelerated electron is focalized on a metallic target made by Mo or W in the case of medical applications, or by Cu, Rh, or another metal in the case of scientific utilization (Figure 3.3a). In turn, the gamma ray sources consist of a certain amount of radioactive isotopes kept in lead or depleted uranium containers (Figure 3.3b).

Regardless of their type, X- and gamma rays interact, at energy beyond the 1.022 MeV pair generation thresholds, by three different mechanisms of which reciprocal contribution depends on the photon energy and the density and mass attenuation coefficient of the material. One of these interactions, the elastic coherent scattering, takes place without any transfer of energy to the exposed body, the incident photons changing only their direction. Therefore, the coherent scattering determines the diffusion of incident photons without any absorption and no energy deposition within the irradiated body.

The coherent scattering cross section σ depends on photon energy ε and absorber atomic number Z following the relation:

$$\sigma_{coh} \sim \frac{Z}{\varepsilon^2} \qquad (3.1)$$

It can be remarked that the probability of coherent interaction decreases with the square photon energy ε and increases with the atomic number Z.

The next mechanism of interaction consists of the photoelectric effect. Opposite to coherent scattering, the photoelectric effect consists of a photon interaction with the atom, the photon transferring its entire energy to a bound electron. As a result, the photon ceases

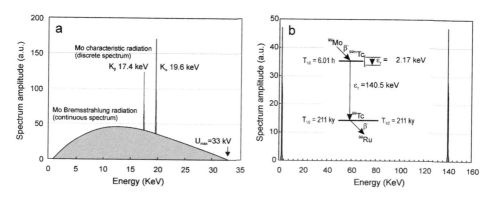

Figure 3.3 The energy spectrum of Mo anode X-ray generator (a) and gamma-ray 99mTc isotopic source (b), both of them intensively used in medicine imaging. The X-ray spectrum consists of Mo X-ray florescence characteristic lines superposed onto the continuum Bremsstrahlung one while the 99mTc spectrum consists of only two discrete lines, the 2.17 keV being totally absorbed in material so that only the 104.5 keV one can be utilized on medical imaging.

existing, its energy, minus the binding energy, being transferred to an electron usually called a photoelectron which is ejected from the atom. It should be remarked that, due to the conservation of momentum, in the case of the photoelectric effect, the photons interact only with bound electrons.

Accordingly, between the photoelectron energy e_{ph}, photon energy ε, and ionizing energy E_i there is the following relation:

$$e_{ph} = \varepsilon - E_i \qquad (3.2)$$

As photoelectrons are charged particles with rest mass, they interact with the atoms of the irradiated medium, transferring by a finite number of ionization and excitation acts their entire energy. Therefore, by the photoelectric effect, the irradiated medium receives the entire energy of the incident photon minus the ionizing energy.

The photoelectric effects cross section depends in a rather complex manner on the photon energy and target medium atomic number:

$$\sigma_{ph} \sim Z^a / \varepsilon^b \qquad (3.3)$$

where a varies between 3 and 4 and b decreases from 7/2 for energies lower than the electron rest mass of 511 keV to 1/2 for energies well above this value.

Accordingly, the probability of photoelectric interaction decreases with the photon energy but remains, in a certain measure, strongly dependent on the atomic number Z. For this reason, lead ($Z = 82$) and depleted uranium ($Z = 92$) are the best materials for shielding high-energy X- and gamma rays.

The Compton effect or inelastic scattering is the last mechanism of photon interaction with matter. It is worth mentioning that the photons interact by the Compton effect with free or almost free electrons so that the cross section is proportional to the atomic number. At the same time, its cross section slowly increases with the energy, reaching a maximum of around 80–100 keV, and then gradually decreases.

$$\sigma_C \sim Z \cdot F(\varepsilon) \qquad (3.4)$$

In Compton inelastic scattering, the photons partially transfer their energy to electrons, resulting in scatted photons caring a fraction of incident photons energy and recoils electron, transporting the difference. For the energies of the order of keV, the differential cross section is almost identical for the forward and backward scattering, but at energies of the order of MeV, the forward scattering becomes dominant.

Therefore, by Compton scattering, the photons partially transfer their energy by means of recoil electrons, changing direction at the same time.

As all these three mechanisms coexist, the interaction of photons with matter is described as a global cross section equal to the sum of the individual cross sections (3.1), (3.3), and (3.4), i.e.:

$$\sigma = \sigma_{coh} + \sigma_{ph} + \sigma_C \qquad (3.5)$$

By passing through material, due to all mentioned interaction, a beam of photons is attenuated either by diffusion, or by absorption. This process is parameterized and characterized by the linear attenuation coefficient (LAC) μ, defined as the probability of interaction on the unity of path and equal to the global cross section multiplied by the number of atoms in the unit of volume n expressed by means of density ρ and mass number A:

$$\mu = n\sigma = \frac{\rho}{A} N_A \sigma = \rho \mu_m \tag{3.6}$$

where N_A represents Avogadro's number and μ_m defines the mass attenuation coefficient (MAC) of which values are independent of the material density but depend on the material atomic number and photon energy.

To illustrate this, in Figure 3.4 we have reproduced the LAC energy dependency of two main components of the human body, soft tissue and bones, whose representation on radiography and CT is essential in evidencing the anatomic formations. Due to the fact that bone tissue is richer in Ca whose atomic number equal to 20 is significantly higher than the soft tissue atomic number of about 7.8, the bone LAC appears significantly higher than that of soft tissue especially at photon energies lower than 60–80 keV. On the other hand, it should be remarked that bone tissue has an average density of 1.9 g/cm³, about twice as high as those of soft tissue whose average density of 1.05 makes it more transparent with respect to the bone. This peculiarity allows evidencing in mammography of micro-calcification at early stages of mammary cancer.

At the same time, for X-ray energy below 500 keV, Compton scattering represents the dominant mechanism of interaction. As the Compton scattering cross section is proportional to the atomic number Z, it results that for these energies, LAC, which in a first approximation

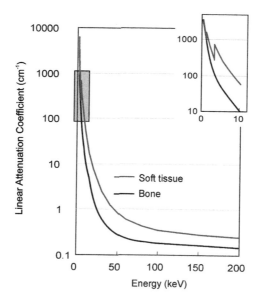

Figure 3.4 Energy dependency of the linear attenuation coefficients (LAC) of soft tissue and bone; the latter, due to the presence of Ca, shows higher values. The existing gap between soft tissue and bone LAC represents the radiological contrast which is well evidenced in radiographies. The inset illustrates the Ca absorption edge which corresponds to the K atomic shell. LAC based on National Institute for Standard and Technology (NIST) data [8].

is proportional to the product of density with the atomic to mass number ratio, becomes, for light elements such as those which compose the soft tissues, dependent only on the absorbent density, well expressed in the case of CT investigations. Since LAC has a good correlation to the type of material/tissue present, the images obtained offer a fair approximation to the types of tissues present.

Under these circumstances, a pencil beam of X- or gamma rays is attenuated by following the well-known Beer–Lambert–Bouguer law:

$$I(x) = I_0 e^{-\mu x} \tag{3.7}$$

where $I(x)$ represents the intensity of the emergent beam of photons, I_0 represents the intensity of the incident beam, and x represents the path length of the beam through the irradiated object.

The pencil beam constraint was included to count only the photons which didn't interact with the material and which are the main component of radiographic and CT images. In real cases, the transited, non-interacting photons which carry the information of the internal structure of the object are superposed onto scattered photons which represent the background void of any information. This peculiarity plays a crucial role in the formation of radiographic images, so that the lower the scattered background, the richer the information represented by the final radiographic image.

Radiographic Image

A radiographic image, as mentioned before, is created by the fraction of an X- or gamma ray beam which, projected toward an object, passes through it without interacting and is captured by an appropriate detector which could be a radiographic film or a solid-state detector. As the process of interaction, in the case of both X- and gamma rays, is parameterized by the LAC, the radiographic image represents the 2D projection of the LAC 3D distribution function of the object.

The final radiographic image, i.e., that which appears on radiographic film or on the CT monitor, represents the results of the interaction of the primary radiant image consisting of the emerging beam of photons with the detector. This means that both the characteristics of the radiant image and those of the detector will contribute to the quality of the final radiography.

In the case of inhomogeneous objects, LAC varies within the object so that Equation 3.7 becomes:

$$I(r) = I_0 e^{-\int \mu(x,y,z)dr} \tag{3.8}$$

where the integral is performed along the X- or gamma rays' path through the object.

The formation of the radiographic image is illustrated in Figure 3.5. Here, it can be observed that the detector simultaneously interacts with the transmitted as well as with the scattered photons. It should be remarked that, while the transmitted photons are attenuated along their path, the scattered ones come from the entire volume. Therefore, only the transmitted photon beam is modulated by means of the object LAC while the information

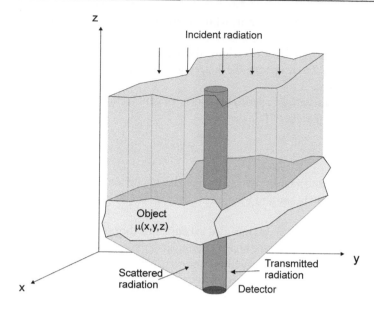

Figure 3.5 The formation of a radiant image in the presence of scattered radiation.

transported by scattered photons is mediated, forming a background. This process is qualitatively described by the following relation:

$$I_{mg}(x,y) \sim \left[I_0 e^{-\int_{z1}^{z2} \mu(x.z.y)dz} + I_{obj} \iiint_V S(x,y,z)dV \right] \tag{3.9}$$

where $I_{mg}(x,y)$ represents the 2D radiographic image as a numeric function whose values vary between 0 (black) and 255 (white); the second term is related to the attenuation of the direct photon beam while the third term describes the incident photon scattering on the whole object.

Equation 3.9 can be rewritten as:

$$I_{mg}(x,y) \sim I_0 e^{-\int_{z1}^{z_2} \mu(x.y.z)dz} (1+R) \tag{3.10}$$

where R represents the contribution of scattered photons to the radiographic image and of which values are around 2.

Equation 3.10 shows with clarity that in the formation of radiographic image, the background consisting of scattered photons plays a significant role. Therefore, the quality of radiographic image is characterized in equal proportion by the contrast of the radiant image and detector spatial resolution. At the same time, the contribution of scattered radiation to the final radiant image depends on the size of the X-rayed body, so the greater the body size, the more significant the background of scattered radiation.

The contrast of the radiant image, called the radiometric contrast, is defined as the difference of the radiant images in the vicinity of a detail characterized by a different LAC (Figure 3.6):

Incident radiation

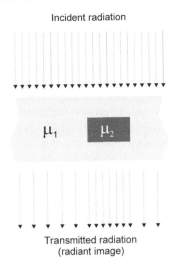

Transmitted radiation
(radiant image)

Figure 3.6 The contrast of a radiant image.

$$C = \frac{I_{mg}(x_1, y_1) - I_{mg}(x_2, y_2)}{I_{mg}(x_1, y_1)} = \frac{e^{-\int_{z_1}^{z_2} \mu(x_1 \cdot y_1 \cdot z)dz} - e^{-\int_{z_1}^{z_2} \mu(x_2 \cdot y_2 \cdot z)dz}}{e^{-\int_{z_1}^{z_2} \mu(x \cdot y \cdot z)dz}(1+R)} \tag{3.11}$$

Which, for two homogenous media with different thickness, becomes $C = \dfrac{1 - e^{\mu \Delta x}}{(1+R)}$ or for two media having different LAC: $C = \dfrac{1 - e^{x \Delta \mu}}{(1+R)}$. In the last case the LAC difference $\Delta \mu$ defines the radiometric contrast. In both cases, the contrast of the radiant image is significantly worsening due to scattered radiation, and this needs different procedures to reduce its influence (see further discussion).

Another aspect related to the presence of scattered radiation concerns the patient surface dose. By considering a detail with a volume x^3 and a LAC differing with the surrounding tissue by a small amount $\Delta \mu$, the patient surface dose D depends on detail size x and X-ray energy E following the relation [9]:

$$D = \mu^t_{m,abs} E \frac{k^2}{\varepsilon}(1+R)\frac{e^{\mu 4t}}{(\Delta \mu)^2}\frac{1}{x^4} \tag{3.12}$$

where $\mu^t_{m,abs}$ represents the mass absorption coefficient of the tissue, μ_t is the tissue LAC, and ε represents the detector efficiency.

This simple model shows that, in order to diminish the patient risk, the radiometric contrast $\Delta \mu$ should be maximized while the contribution of scattered radiation should be significantly reduced as well as the exposure time.

The radiometric contrast $\Delta \mu$ could be increased by choosing X- or gamma rays of low energy where the photoelectric effect has a significant contribution, but this is achieved with an increased opacity which needs a longer exposure.

In turn, the contribution of scattered radiation can be reduced either by using multihole collimators as in the case of cone beam geometry or slit collimators and translational exposure in the case of fan beam exposure.

A multihole collimator is a device consisting of an array of hollow cells formed between thin vertical walls. The cell can be hexagonal, round, or square. The walls are made of high atomic number elements such as tungsten or lead. Depending on the reciprocal orientation of the cell axis, multihole collimators could be convergent, parallel, or divergent with respect to the radiation source (Figure 3.7). To reduce the scattered radiation, the multihole collimators are placed tightly in front of the detector.

The parameter which characterizes the multihole collimators is the contrast gain C_G which defines the contrast of the radiant image at the exit of the collimator:

$$C_G = \left(1 + \frac{R_G}{R}\right)C \tag{3.13}$$

where $R_G = \dfrac{h}{D}$ defines the collimator parameter equal to the ratio between the collimator thickness h and distance between cell walls D while R represents the ratio of scattered and transmitted radiation according to Equation 3.10.

Depending on the collimator parameter R_G, their use can compensate up to 90% of the loss of radiant image contrast due to the scattered radiation. At the same time, a small per cent of incident radiation can penetrate the inner walls, contributing in this way to image unsharpness.

On the other hand, the collimators, depending on the material they are made of as well as on the energy of the X- or gamma rays, can absorb up to 95% of the incident photons, which raises the problem of patient exposure to high ionizing radiation. In this regard, to achieve a balance between patient exposure and image quality, the collimators are designed in function of X- or gamma ray energy. In the case of X-rays with energies up to 150 keV, the most appropriate are the low-energy high-spatial definition collimators with thin inner walls and small holes, while in the case of higher energy the inner walls are thicker and holes larger, with a corresponding diminution of spatial resolution.

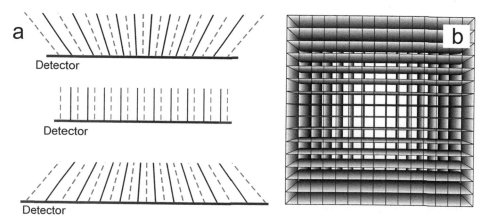

Figure 3.7 The schematic representation of different configurations of collimators (a) as well as a general view of a parallel walls mutihole collimator (b).

In all cases, a supplementary diminution of the patient irradiation can be achieved by increasing the X-ray detector efficiency which implies the use of fluorescence intensifying screens [10].

The intensifying screens consist of a thin layer of X-ray fluorescent material which by absorbing X-ray photons emits visible light to which the radiographic films are more sensitive. At present, the most utilized fluorescent materials are REE oxisulphides such as Y_2O_2S:Tb and Gd_2O_2S:Pr or oxibromide such as LaOBr:Tm, which convert about 20% of the energy of incident X- or gamma rays into visible light. Their advantage concerning the patient can be easily understood as, on average, for one X-ray photon absorbed by the screen, there are released about 3,000 visible light photons easily absorbed by the radiographic film, which significantly reduces the patient's absorbed dose [11]. The main drawback of X-ray fluorescence screens is related to the worsening of final image resolution due to the light diffusion within the detector.

The spatial resolution, the second important property of the radiographic image, refers to the capacity of a radiographic system to evidence distinctly near-by objects as well as to represent with accuracy the object contour. In radiographic systems as well as in any imaging system, the resolution depends on how the radiographic image forms as well as on the size of detector elements.

In an ideal case, the radiation source, either an X-ray generator or gamma ray isotopic source, should be as small as possible to reduce the optical penumbra (Figure 3.8). According to the optical path illustrated in Figure 3.8, the radiographic image of a detail Dtl which represents its geometric umbra U_g is flanked by a geometric penumbra P_g that worsens the image by reducing its spatial resolution.

From geometric considerations, the size of geometric penumbra P_g depends on the source dimension S, focal distance d_1, and the gap d_2 between object and detector, as follows:

$$P_G = s\frac{d_2}{d_1} = s(m-1) \tag{3.14}$$

where m represents the magnification $m = \dfrac{d_1 + d_2}{d_1} \geq 1$.

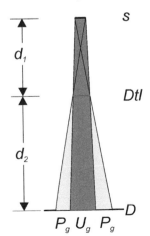

Figure 3.8 The geometric characteristic of an X- or gamma ray radiant image. s: source of radiation (X- or gamma rays), Dtl: detail, D: detector, U_g: geometric umbra, P_g: geometric penumbra.

This simple model shows how to control and reduce the geometric penumbra in order to increase the radiographic image spatial resolution: (a) by decreasing the source diameter S; (b) by reducing the gap d_2 between object and detector; and (c) by increasing the focal length d_1 to keep the magnification as close as possible to the unit. Regarding the last condition, this does not apply for micro-tomography or micro-radiography where the only way to get a significant magnification is to keep the distance d_2 between object and detector as great as possible. In this case, the source diameter S plays an essential role which is why micro-focus X-ray generators or synchrotron radiation [12] are used, where the effective source diameter can be reduced to a few microns.

The radiant image detectors contribute also to the final radiography spatial resolution with its intrinsic unsharpness F related to the size of silver grain in the case of radiographic film or the size of individual light detectors.

Accordingly, by combining the two kinds of unsharpness according to the error composing law:

$$U = \sqrt{P_g^2 + U_d^2} \tag{3.15}$$

where U represents the global unsharpness, $U_d = \dfrac{F}{m}$ is the detector's unsharpness, and F is the detector's intrinsic unsharpness, which in the case of an SSD detector is equal, according to the Nyquist–Whittaker–Shannon theorem [13], to double the detector size.

By taking into account the expression of geometric penumbra (14), the unsharpness of the final radiographic image becomes:

$$U = \frac{F}{m} \sqrt{1 + m^2(m-1)^2 \frac{s^2}{F^2}} \tag{3.16}$$

The graphical representation of this relation illustrates that the main factors which control the unsharpness are source size and magnification (Figure 3.9).

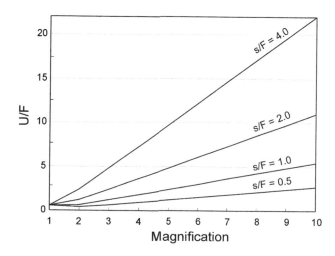

Figure 3.9 The dependence of the total U/F ratio on the magnification for different source s to elemental detector size ratios.

From this point of view, higher resolution can be achieved by using, where possible, point-like radiation sources as well as detectors with the smallest detection units. From this point of view, the radiographic film in which silver halide grains have submicron sizes seems to have, when used without intensifying screens, the best resolution [11].

With the development of SSD, digital radiography is becoming more and more a routine technique which, mainly due to a continuous reduction of individual detector sizes to 50 μm × 50 μm, provides a submillimetric spatial resolution.

The radiographic image, either on film or projected on a PC monitor and printed on polyester foil, represents the final product of a set of operations performed in real time as in the case of digital radiography or after the radiographic film is exposed and then processed. In both cases, the radiography is characterized, as mentioned before, by contrast and spatial resolution. Regardless of the modality by the radiographic image is produced, its spatial resolution significantly depends on a complex chain from radiation source to detector.

The best way to characterize the performance of any X- or gamma ray imaging system consists of the analysis of the spatial frequency spectrum of the final radiographic image. For exemplification, in Figure 3.10 is reproduced an image of a spectral frequency, which in fact can be regarded as a sinusoidal variation of image intensity along a single direction, similar to an ideal curtain. The periodicity of a spatial frequency is expressed in cycles/unit of length, usually cycles/mm. Similar to the spectral characterization of sound or of any other electrical signal by its frequency spectrum, the analysis of any image, regardless of how it was acquired, can be done by means of its spatial frequency spectrum.

Indeed, any image can be expressed as a superposition of a multitude of spatial frequencies covering all directions and of which maximum number of cycles per unit of length defines the image spatial resolution. Therefore, the higher the spatial frequencies, the lower the resulting image unsharpness.

The spatial frequency distribution of an image can be done by the 2D Fourier transform which illustrates the presence of different spatial frequencies. This is illustrated in Figure 3.11

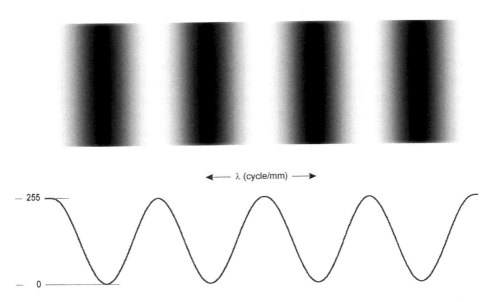

Figure 3.10 Spatial frequency (up) and the corresponding sinusoidal variation of grey hues (down).

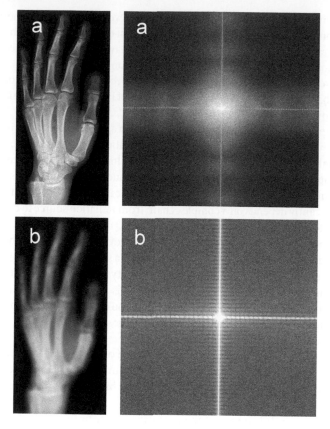

Figure 3.11 Two radiographic images of the right hand with different spatial resolution and the corresponding FFT. The radiography (a) has a better resolution than the radiography (b) well evidenced in the FFT spectra by an increased presence of higher frequencies visible around the centre of the FFT spectrum (radiography courtesy of Mikael Häggström).

where two radiographic images of the same right hand with different resolutions are accompanied by the corresponding spatial frequencies fast Fourier transform (FFT) spectra. It can be observed that in the case of the low-resolution image, its FFT spectrum presents a narrow maximum in the central zone, different from the FTT spectrum of the high-resolution radiograph, where the central maximum is significantly extended, attesting to the presence of higher spatial frequencies.

In order to characterize the final spatial resolution of an imaging instrument such as a radiograph or computed tomography (CT) image, the modulation transfer function (MTF) represents one of the best descriptors [14]. It represents the frequency distribution of the response of an imaging system to monotonously increasing spatial frequencies. As the radiological imaging systems are shift invariant, i.e., when the input is a sinusoid function, as in the case of spatial frequencies, the output will be also a sinusoid function. Due to the fact that geometric penumbra and finite detector size reduce the modulation depth as frequency increases, the MTF can be defined for a sine wave spatial frequency as the modulation depth of the radiographic image relative to what is entering the imaging system:

$$MTF(\xi) = \frac{A(\xi)_{max} - A(\xi)_{min}}{A(\xi)_{max} + A(\xi)_{min}} \tag{3.17}$$

where $A(\xi)_{max}$ and $A(\xi)_{min}$ are the maximum and minimum amplitudes of the spatial frequency ξ.

As the difference $\Delta A(\xi) = A(\xi)_{max} - A(\xi)_{min}$ represents the image contrast corresponding to spatial frequency ξ, the MTF could be regarded as the contrast distribution over the considered domain of spatial frequencies.

The MTF can be determined experimentally by means of sinusoidal (Figure 3.12a) or opaque bar (Figure 3.12b) target of which sizes monotonously decreases. In both cases, the higher frequencies are firstly attenuated. As mentioned before, it is obvious that the higher the frequency whose contrast appears on MTF, the higher the spatial resolution of the considered radiographic system.

By the 1980s, radiographies were done by using radiographic film, an adaptation for the high-energy X- and gamma ray of the photographic film. Radiographic film plays the role of a converter and recorder of the radiant image by transforming it into a long-lasting optical image which reproduces with a certain degree of fidelity the spatial distribution of the intensity of transmitted radiation which forms the radiant image. Unlike the photographic film, the radiographic film has a radiation-sensitive emulsion, i.e., the true radiation detector, on both sides of a transparent base, actually polyester [9]. This configuration increases by a factor of two the efficiency of X- or gamma rays, reducing the patient irradiation accordingly.

The parameter which quantitatively describes the radiographic image as it appears on film is the optical density (D) defined as the decimal logarithm of the light transmission through the film (transmittance) according to:

$$D \equiv \lg T = \lg \frac{I_0}{I} \tag{3.18}$$

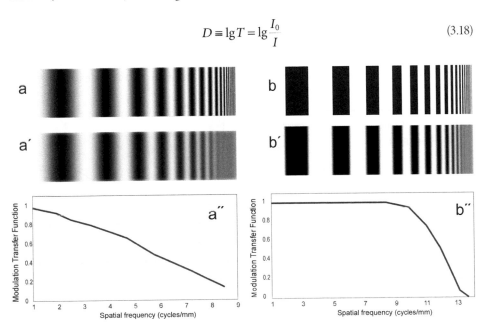

Figure 3.12 A sinusoidal (a) and a bar pattern (b), their images produced by an X-ray imaging system (a′) and (b′) and the corresponding modulation transfer function (a″) and (b″). In both cases, the higher frequencies are gradually attenuated.

where T is the transmittance, and I_0 and I are the intensity of incident and transmitted light.

The logarithmic scale was chosen because the human eye responds, according to the Weber–Fechner laws [15], logarithmically to the variation of the light intensity.

The optical density can be correlated with the exposure X of the incident on film of the X- or gamma ray photons by means of the Nutting law [9,16]:

$$D = 0.434\,\bar{a}\,N(1 - e^{-\bar{a}kX})$$

(3.19)

where $\bar{a}$ is the average area of silver grain after the film was processed, N is the area density of silver halide grains of unexposed film, and k is a constant which depends on the probability of interaction between the incident photons and the silver halide grains.

The Nutting law predicts a saturation exponential dependency of the optical density on the exposure, very close to the real one as described by the characteristic (sensitometric) curve illustrated in Figure 3.13. The existence of a sigmoid dependence between optical density and exposure, as both the Nutting law and experimental sensitometric curves illustrate, proves the absence of a true proportionality between optical density and exposure which, in its turn, represents a source of systematic errors. This is true especially at both extremities of the characteristic curve which correspond to under- and overexposed sections respectively (Figure 3.13). Moreover, even the central part of the curve which defines the range of diagnostic densities can be considered approximately linear allowing rather a qualitative estimation of the X- and gamma ray attenuation. To this should be added a relatively limited dynamic range of exposure corresponding to a diagnostic density range which varies between 25 and 50, while the range of transmitted radiation exposure can vary between 1 and 100, or even more. This behaviour is due to the fact that: (a) a silver halide grain to be further converted into a silver grain during the chemical processing of the exposed film needs, according to Gurney and Mott's theory [16], more X- or gamma ray quanta to interact with which explains the existence of the underexposed section; (b) the amount of silver halide grains is limited so, with the increasing of exposure, the number of unexposed grains is exhausted which explains the overexposure section where in fact a saturation takes place.

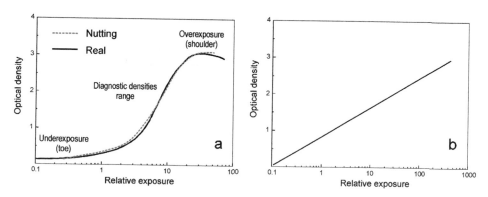

Figure 3.13 A comparisons between the exposure diagram of a radiographic film (a) and of an SSD utilized in digital radiography (b). The diagram (a) has a characteristic S shape which appears when a saturation exponential dependency is logarithmically represented. In the case of diagram (b), due to multiple readouts the saturation does not appear and the optical density depends linearly on relative exposure. It can be remarked also the difference between the relative exposure dynamic range of radiographic film (a) and SSD (b).

Regardless of these limitations, the film radiography, due to the micron sizes of silver grains, has a spatial resolution never attained by the actual digital radiography. Moreover, film radiographies, due to a remarkable physical resilience, have unlimited conservation time, which makes them ideal archive objects with physical support.

With the development of digital radiography in the last decades, some of the inherent limitations of film radiography such as the nonlinear response of radiographic film as well as its long and complex processing necessary to obtain final radiographies have been overcome. Indeed, the actual image detectors, image plate or photodiode array, permitted obtaining in real-time radiographic images whose quality concerning spatial resolution is comparable or even better than the classic film radiographies.

To this it should be added the perfect linear response of the imaging detectors to exposure as well as the possibility of using a dual-energy technique which permits the simultaneous determination of both local density and the effective atomic number for any part of an investigated body or to virtually separate soft tissue from bones which significantly improves the diagnostic quality.

The linear response to exposition in the case of digital radiography is due to the way image radiation detectors respond to incident X- or gamma rays. Unlike the radiographic film, in the case of digital radiography, the X-rays are detected by means of the electric charge generated in a solid state. This can be done directly as in the case of photo-conducting layer technology (usually a thin layer of amorphous Se), or indirectly, by means of a photodiode coupled to a scintillator material such as CsI:Tl or Gd_2O_2S [17]. As the readout can be reduced to a few times per second, the risk of saturation, inherent to radiographic films, does not exist providing a dynamic range greater than 5500 (Figure 3.13b).

These detectors can be disposed by forming an image plate consisting of up to 2400×2400 individual detectors of size 50×50 μm providing a spatial resolution up to 10 line pairs/mm. This is the configuration used in cone beam geometry currently used in medical digital radiography. The same types of detectors can be arranged by forming linear arrays consisting of one or a few parallel sets of detectors by forming a final array consisting of 4096×128 individual detectors of 48×48 μm at a spatial resolution slightly higher than 100 line pairs/mm making the translational radiography one of its major beneficiaries.

Computed Tomography

CT is the second medical imaging technique based on the transmission of X-rays. Unlike radiography, which generates 2D images of the projection of the investigated body, without any information concerning the spatial distribution of organs, CT reconstructs the distribution function of the LAC in a section of the investigated object [18]. By adding more consecutive CT images it becomes possible to obtain a true 3D image of the considered body, illustrating the spatial distribution of different organs and tissues with a millimetre precision and accuracy.

For this, instead of the cone beam geometry used in radiography, in CT a thin fan beam is used so that the contribution of scatter radiation is significantly reduced. In this way, Equation 3.10 becomes:

$$I(x,y) \sim I_0 e^{\int_{z_1}^{z_2} \mu(x,y,z)dz} \tag{3.20}$$

Here, the investigated body is represented by its 3D LAC distribution function $\mu(x,y,z)$ whose value appears as an integrand. The value of the integral can be experimentally determined in a section x0y of the investigated object, by means of the natural logarithm of the ratio of incident to transmitted X-rays, for any angle φ' along any axis x' (Figure 3.14):

$$\lambda_\varphi(x') = \ln\frac{I_0}{I} = \int_S^D \mu(x,y)dy' = \int_{-\infty}^{+\infty}\int_{-\infty}^{+\infty} \mu[x,y]\delta\left(x\cos\varphi + y\sin\varphi - x'\right)dx\,dy \qquad (3.21)$$

where $\lambda_\varphi(x')$ represents the Radon transform [19] of the 2D $\mu[x,y]$ LAC function. It worth mentioning that the Radon transform for a certain value of the angle φ represents the projection of the $\mu[x,y]$ function along the direction x' so that the Radon transform can be regarded as the totality of projection of the LAC function.

Conversely, once the Radon transform is acquired, the reconstruction of the initial LAC function can be done by applying the inverse Radon transform:

$$\mu[x,y] = -\frac{1}{2\pi^2}\lim_{x\to 0}\int_\varepsilon^\infty \frac{1}{x'}\int_0^{2\pi} \frac{d\lambda_\varphi(x')}{dl}\,d\varphi\,dx' \qquad (3.22)$$

In this way, the $\mu[x,y]$ function can be recalculated by solving the inverse problem, i.e., recalculating a function from its projection [18]. While radiography, regardless of whether

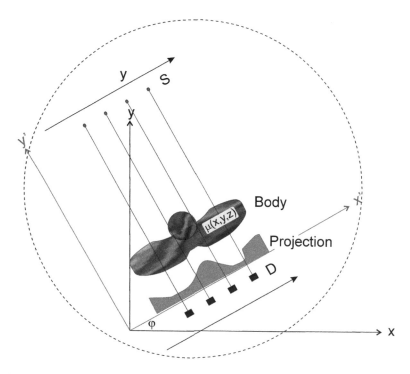

Figure 3.14 Generation of the projection of the investigated body described by its 2D function of the LAC.

it is radiographic film or digital, in fact represents an analogical representation of the LAC projection. In the case of CT, to solve the inverse problem it needs an elaborated mathematical procedure which can be done by using powerful computers. It should be remarked that in the reconstruction process, which is an essentially digital operation, it is implied that the investigated section is virtually divided into a great number of identical elemental volumes, voxels, usually 256×256 or 512×512, each of them supposed to be homogenous so that they can be characterized by single values of CAL. In this way, the reconstructed tomography will consist of a matrix of 256×256 or 512×512 different values, each of them corresponding to the corresponding voxel.

Accordingly, the first step in obtaining a CT consist of the acquisition of the linear projection which is done by rotating a high-output small focal spot X-ray generator around the body, In this way, the transmitted radiation is detected by a set of detectors disposed on a circular gantry which surrounds both patient and X-ray source (Figure 3.15). As detectors form a circular array, their output is rescaled to reconstruct a linear projection, as illustrated in Figure 3.14. Their number and size play a major role in the quality of reconstructed LAC function, because on this depends the extent to which the final CT images reproduce with fidelity the anatomic structures. Here, the maximum spatial resolution is related, as in the case of digital radiography, to the detector size as, the minimum thickness of evidenced detail, could no smaller than its projection on the two neighbouring detectors [13]. By considering that to each detector corresponds a pixel of the reconstructed image, the maximum spatial frequency which could be present in the final reconstructed image corresponds, as mentioned before, to the double detector width, this frequency called theNyquist frequency being equal to 0.5 cycle/pixel.

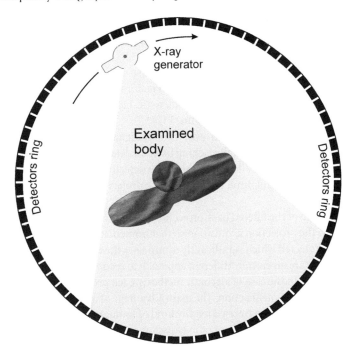

Figure 3.15 The reciprocal disposition of the X-ray generator, examined body, and detectors for a fourth-generation CT. A black dot marks the position of the X-ray generator focal spot.

For a given orientation of the X-ray generator, the outputs of each detector are recorded by forming a series of numeric data which, after being corrected for difference in detector output, are converted, by means of fan-to-parallel rebinning, into parallel beam projection. The use of a significant number of identical detectors determines the sampling of LAS projection to be equal to the individual detector width. For a good reconstruction, the number of projections could be as high as possible, but in real cases, their number varies between 360 and 720. To collect them, the X-ray source should effectuate a complete rotation around the examined body, as illustrated in Figure 3.15.

Once a complete set of projections has been acquired, the next stage consists of reconstructing the LAC distribution function of its projections. Instead of using the inverse Radon transform, which is a tedious process, at present time there are in use two methods for approximately solving the inverse problem, i.e., filtered back projection (a Fourier transform-based technique) [20] and algebraic reconstruction [21]. In both cases, a 2D LAC $\mu[x,y]$ distribution function is reconstructed from a set of 1D projections which really represents a remarkable achievement of applied mathematics.

The filtered back projection technique is based on the central slice theorem according to which the Fourier transform of a linear projection of a function represents a section in the Fourier transform of that function, in our case the LAC $\mu[x,y]$ distribution. Accordingly, this technique implies the back projection of each previously acquired projection convoluted with a digital filter whose purpose consists of amplifying high spatial frequencies up to a maximum cut-off whose value is determined, as mentioned before, by the detector width [20,21]. In this way, regardless of the filter type, the contribution of low spatial frequencies that determine the presence of blurring in final reconstructed CT images is significantly reduced. At the same time, the existence of a cut-off frequency does not allow the presence of spatial frequencies higher than the Nyquist one which represent only noise likely to alter the quality of the reconstructed images. For comparison, in Figure 3.16 there are reproduced two digital filters, Ramachandran–Lakshminarayanan [22] (Figure 3.16a) and Shepp–Logan [23] (Figure 3.16b) together with their frequency response. Here it can be remarked that in the case of the Shepp–Logan filter, the amplification factor tends to zero at higher spatial frequencies. But both filters have the same characteristic, i.e., negative values where abrupt changes of projection magnitudes occur (Figure 3.17).

The use of filters is absolutely imperative as, without digital filtering, the resulting reconstructed images are unclear, totally lacking in small details (Figure 3.18). In the case of filtered back projection, the smaller the width of the detectors, the more accurate are the reconstructed images, so that, at limit, the filtered back projection merges with the inverse Radon transform.

The main advantage of the filtered back projection consists of a quasi-simultaneous reconstruction with the projection acquisition so that immediately when a projection is acquired it is back projected which significantly diminishes the computing time.

Algebraic methods are an entirely different approach to reconstructing images. Unlike the filtered back projection, in the case of algebraic methods, each projection is stored separately before being used for the reconstruction. The main advantage of algebraic methods consists in their universality, i.e., they can be used for any kind of tomography techniques, either transmissive or emissive such as single photon emission computed tomography (SPECT) or PET. They also offer a nice decoupling between the model, i.e., the final reconstructed tomography image and the reconstruction algorithms. This modularity allows a better parallelism of the different components of algebraic reconstruction to optimize the computing code as well.

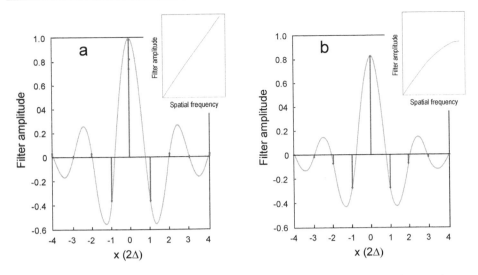

Figure 3.16 The Ramachandran–Lakshminarayanan (a) and Shepp–Logan (b) filters. Grey continuous line: analytical form, red vertical line: digital variant use for filtering. The insets reproduce the corresponding spatial frequency amplification.

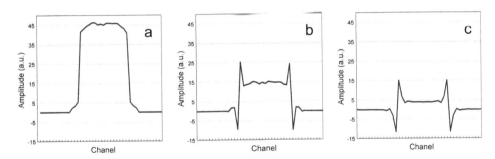

Figure 3.17 The results of digital filtration of a projection of a homogenous cylindrical object (a) performed by Ramachandran–Lakshminarayanan (b) and Shepp–Logan (c) filters. Note the negative component of filtered projection which corresponds to abrupt changes of projection values.

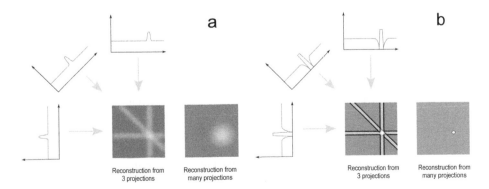

Figure 3.18 The reconstruction of the same circular object by unfiltered (a) and filtered (b) back projection methods. In the first case, the contour is blurred as for this method the contour varied following a 1/r dependency, which is not the case of filtered back projection.

Algebraic algorithms assume the LAC of each voxel to be initially unknown which means a system of linear algebraic equations is needed in order to calculate these starting from the recorded projections.

By particularizing the Radon transform for a discrete distribution of voxels, it results, according to [21], in a system of 256×256 or 512×512 (more than 10^5) linear equations:

$$\lambda_\varphi(x') = \sum_{i=1}^{n} A_i(x', \varphi) \mu_i[x, y] \tag{3.23}$$

where $A_i(x', \varphi)$, called the system matrix, describes with what probability a voxel i contributes to the projection $\lambda(x')$, a contribution equal to the path length of the projection through the considered voxel. It is obvious that for each orientation φ and position x' the coefficients $A_i(x', \varphi)$ will take different values which can be calculated once for the entire system of projections.

In this way, the problem of reconstruction of LAC on projections can be reduced to solving a system of more than 10^5 equations, which is almost impossible, taking into account that, among other things, each projection is affected by experimental uncertainties. For this reason, as in the case of filtered back projection, it seeking an approximate solution of the system (23). In this case, the solution consists of gradually adjusting the values of LAC of each voxel, computing each time the resulting projections until, between the initial set of projections and the recalculated ones with adjusted values of individual LAC, the difference, by minimizing an error function, satisfies a certain criterion of likelihood. At this moment, the LAC of each voxel as resulting from the last iteration could be considered the final reconstructed LAC distribution function within the considered section, i.e., the reconstructed tomographic image.

Therefore, reconstructions with algebraic methods consist of two main steps: the construction of the system matrix $A_i(x', \varphi)$ and the computation of the unknown LAC μ_i of the considered section. This decoupling offers a great deal of flexibility, because almost any kind of reconstruction can be done as long as a good model is available for it.

Besides the fact that algebraic methods can be used for both transmissive and emissive computed tomography, when constructing the system matrix, different sources for errors can also be considered and included in the model, something not possible with the filtered back projection method.

Scintigraphy

The scintigraphic method was designed to display the spatial 2D or 3D distribution of radiopharmaceutics inside the body in order to evidence the functionality of internal organs such as the heart, lung, thyroid, or liver, or to evidence different tumoral formations.

In its initial 2D variant, the scintigraphy, somehow similar to radiography, generated a 2D projection of the real 3D distribution function of gamma rays emitting medicinal radiocompounds fixed in an organ or a tissue. Unlike radiography, scintigraphy represents, as mentioned before, an emissive medical imaging technique, as the source of radiation is created inside the patient's body by administrating intravenously a radioactive tracer with affinity for a certain organ or tissue.

The fact that the source of radiation has a solid volume determined the creation of a specialized type of detector able to select from the radiations emitted in all directions only those which could generate a true 2D projection.

This can be done either using a source of gamma rays and detectors sensitive to the position of incident photons such as the Anger (gamma) camera [24] or a set of two opposite and in-coincidence detectors for the 511 keV annihilation photons as in the case of PET [25].

The gamma camera represents the central part of any scintigraphy imaging system. It consists of a large and flat scintillator monocrystal, usually NaI(Tl) with a great efficiency in detecting gamma rays optically coupled on one face with an array of photomultiplier tubes and a multihole collimator on the other (Figure 3.19a).

NaI(Tl) was chosen as it converts about 13% of the energy of absorbed gamma photons into luminous scintillations of 415 nm wavelength, prone to be further amplified by appropriate devices such as photomultiplier tubes or avalanche photodiodes. Moreover, the number of scintillation photons generated by NaI(Tl) with a time constant of 230 ns is proportional to the total amount of energy released within the crystal by gamma photons. This permits counting rates between 10^4 and 10^5 counts per second, each count corresponding to a detected gamma photon.

As the quantum noise is equal to the square root of the number of detected photons, a high counting rate results in an increased signal-to-noise ratio and thus, a higher quality of scintigraphic images.

As presented before, at energies below 1,022 keV, the X- or gamma ray photons release their energy by Compton and photoelectric effects. The energy released by the photoelectric

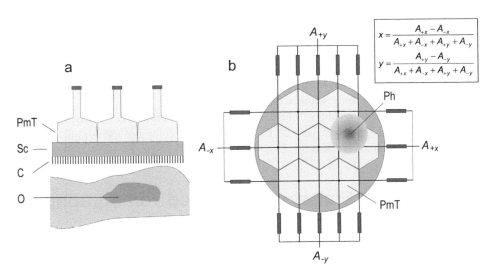

$$x = \frac{A_{+x} - A_{-x}}{A_{+x} + A_{-x} + A_{+y} + A_{-y}}$$

$$y = \frac{A_{+y} - A_{-y}}{A_{+x} + A_{-x} + A_{+y} + A_{-y}}$$

Figure 3.19 The schematic representation of acquisition of a scintigraphic image (a) by using an Anger (gamma) camera with seven hexagonal photomultiplier tubes (b). The inset illustrated how the position of the incident photon on the scintillator crystal is determined by processing in coincidence the amplitudes of signals generated by each of seven photomultiplier tubes. O: the organ containing radiopharmaceutical; C: multihole collimator; Sc: scintillator crystal; PmT: photomultiplier tube. Black rectangles represent the resistor whose values allow recalculating the position of the incident photon (Ph) with respect to the scintillator crystal. The area covered by scintillation photons generated by the incident gamma photon is represented by a small greyish circle with darker center.

effect is equal to the photon energy minus a small amount consumed to ionize the target atoms. In contrast, the energy corresponding to recoil electrons generated by the Compton effect cannot be greater than a fraction of $E_\gamma \Big/ m_e c^2$ from the energy of incident photons, thus discriminating between them and the scattered photons which contribute to the image unsharpness. This is another advantage of using proportional type detectors such as NaI(Tl).

The photomultiplier tubes have a hexagonal, seldom square, shape to cover as much as possible the entire NaI(Tl) crystal. Depending on the crystal diameter, the number of photomultipliers varies between 7 and 91 for diameters between 2.5 and 7.5 cm, so the higher the number, the lower the diameter. All photomultiplier tubes are interconnected via a coincidence circuit following a certain arrangement to code the position of the incident photon on the crystal (Figure 3.19b) with an uncertainty varying between 0.5 and 1.2 cm. It is worth mentioning, for each gamma ray photon which interacts with the crystal, the sum of signals produced by each photomultiplier is proportional to the amount of energy released by photons. This so-called z signal permits discrimination between the energy released by direct and scattered photons.

The third main component of a gamma camera is represented by a multihole collimator, which, depending on its configuration, can magnify, keep as it is, or compress the field of view (Figure 3.7a). The collimator should be considered, as in the case of radiography, the main focussing component of any gamma camera as it allows, with a certain degree of uncertainty, the detection of those photons which by forming a paralleled beam, generate with accuracy the 2D projection of the 3D distribution of activity concentration within the investigated organ or tissue.

It should be pointed out that the final resolution of a gamma camera is controlled by more parameters concerning collimator geometry such as hole sizes and wall thickness, the distance between the object and the collimator's surface as well as crystal intrinsic resolution. Under these circumstances, the better spatial resolution is of the order of a few mm, monotonously increasing with the source-collimator distance up to 1 cm and more. For this reason, the images generated by a gamma camera have a lesser clarity than those obtained by transmissive radiography and computed tomography.

In this way, the gamma or Anger camera represents the most utilized device to generate plane scintigraphic images which, with the development of the computed tomography technique, are the main image detectors for SPECT.

Single Photon Emission Computed Tomography

SPECT represents an advanced medicine imaging method able to provide real 3D imaging illustrating the distribution of the activity concentration of certain radionuclides attached to radiopharmaceuticals targeting specific organs in order to evidence their functionality. Moreover, SPECT permits a whole-body examination during a single session, although, unlike conventional radiography and CT, the exposure to radiation continues until the radiopharmaceutical is completely metabolized and the attached radionuclide is eliminated.

As a tomography method, SPECT permits the reconstruction of a 3D distribution function of activity concentration from its projection obtained by gamma camera. Similar to the classic CT, this is done by acquiring more projection uniformly distributed around the investigated body. This is done by a gantry which contains one to three gamma cameras and which rotates around the examined body in steps of three to six degrees until a compete rotation of 360° is achieved (Figure 3.20). Because the reconstruction accuracy depends on the signal quality provided by each camera, the greater the number of gamma cameras, the higher the quality of the reconstructed images. At the same time, the simultaneous use of more gamma cameras reduces proportionally the acquisition time increasing the accuracy in representing the tissue shape by reducing the influence of patient motion.

A special case is represented by electrocardiogram gated SPECT when the heart is perfused with a radiotracer. Accordingly, the final tomography which illustrates the myocardium functionality allows the detection of myocardial infractions or evidencing the ischemic region caused by a coronary artery disease.

Gamma cameras as well as other emissive imaging techniques are characterized by a significantly lower spatial resolution, no better than 1 cm. Moreover, the presence of radioactive material within the patient's body requires as low as possible radiopharmaceutical which at their turn determines increased level of quantum noises. Combined with a limited spatial resolution, SPECT images are less qualitative than the transmissive CT ones. On the other hand, SPECT provides functional 3D images of the investigated organ, similar to PET and functional NMR.

The lower resolution of gamma camera projections as well as their reduced number with respect to CT makes the reconstruction task difficult so that the algebraic reconstruction techniques such as Monte Carlo-based reconstruction or convolutional neural network furnish better results [26]. Given the progress of artificial intelligence, the last approach appears the most promising for future developments of SPECT as well as PET.

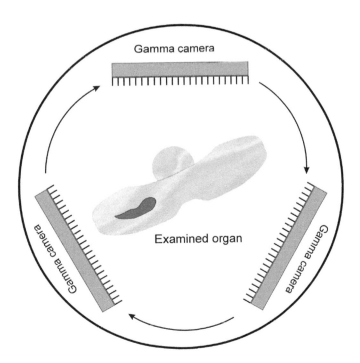

Figure 3.20 The reciprocal disposition of the gamma camera and examined body in a multiple-detector SPECT.

Because the sources of radiation are inside the body, the gamma rays are attenuated by the neighbouring tissues until being detected. The attenuation, which grows with the radiation path within the body, induces errors in the reconstructed images. This is well illustrated in Figure 3.20 where the gamma ray path significantly varies for different positions of the gamma camera with respect to the body. The influence of inner absorption can be reduced in a certain measure by using two gamma cameras oppositely disposed with respect to the body or by extracting the information concerning the gamma-ray path from a CT image synchronously acquired. In spite of improving the quality of the SPECT image, the use of a CT increases the effective dose of radiation administered to the patient, raising the risk of stochastic effects.

The main radionuclides used in SPECT are those which emit gamma rays with a minimum contribution of beta rays, given their reduced path and corresponding higher linear transfer of energy (Table 3.1). In this regard, ^{99m}Tc appears to be the most promising as it represents a metastable state of ^{99}Tc which decays by an isomeric transition without any accompanying charged radiation.

Excepting the ^{67}Ga which can be used in the form of citrate or nitrate owing to its capacity to localize within the body, and ^{201}Tl which is an analogue to potassium, the other radionuclides currently used in SPECT are attached to complex organic molecules that show affinity for some specific organs.

Positron Emission Tomography

PET represents another emissive tomographic image technique intensively used in reconstituting the distribution function of the activity concentration of β^- emitting radionuclides in selected organs or tissues to evidence their functionality.

PET differs from SPECT by the manner in which the projection of radiopharmaceutic-marked organ or tissue is produced. In the case of SPECT, this is done by using multihole collimators and massive NaI(Tl) scintillator crystals for focalization. In the case of PET, instead of collimators, the focalization is done by detecting in coincidence the two 511 keV annihilation photons generated when a positron interacts with an electron (Figure 3.21). This

Table 3.1 The Commonly Used Radioisotopes in SPECT

Radioisotope	γ-Ray Energy (keV)	Half-Life	Decay Mode	Production
^{67}Ga	90.2 to 300.2	3.3 d	ec to ^{67}Zn	^{68}Zn(p, 2n)^{67}Ga
^{99m}Tc	140.5	6.00 h	Isomeric transition to ^{99}Tc	^{100}Mo(p,2n)^{99m}Tc
^{123}I	159	13.22 h	ec to ^{123}Te	^{124}X(p,2n)^{123}I
^{133}Xe	80.9	5.24 d	β^- to ^{133}Cs	^{235}U fission
^{201}Tl	69 to 80	70.2 h	ec to ^{201}Hg	^{201}Hg(p,n)^{201}Tl, ^{202}Hg(p, 2n)^{201}Tl, ^{204}Hg(p, 4n)^{201}Tl,

Note: ec stands for internal conversion

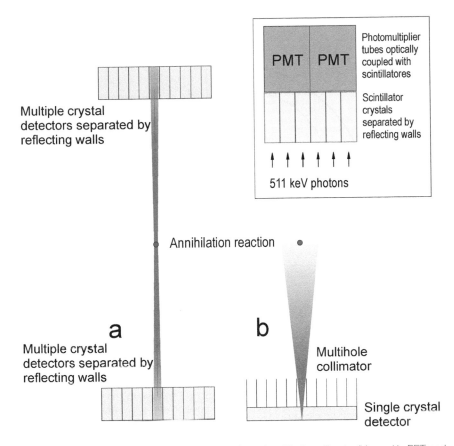

Figure 3.21 The difference between the electronic (a) and multihole collimator (b) used in PET and SPECT respectively. The inset illustrates the multicrystal detector utilized to collimate the annihilation photons.

is possible as, instead of using a gamma camera provided with a massive scintillator crystal and a multihole collimator, PET devices are provided with a multitude of individual detectors disposed in opposite directions and coupled in coincidence to detect only photons generated by the annihilation of the same positron (Figure 3.22). Although the NaI(Tl) scintillator was intensively used in the past decades, new rare earth elements orthosilicates such as Gd_2SiO_5 or Lu_2SiO_5 showed better efficiency and time resolution which recommended them as the future scintillators for SPECT and especially for PET.

Moreover, the positron emitting radioisotopes currently used in PET are isotopes of elements which enter in the composition of living tissue, being perfectly compatible with them (Table 3.2). Therefore, they can be included in a great diversity of molecules whose role is essential in cell metabolism. Among them, ^{18}F seems to be the most convenient as on one hand it has the longest half-life time of about 110 min and can be easily attached to glucose by replacing a normal hydroxyl group in the glucose molecule by forming the fluorodeoxyglucose which acts as a glucose substitute. Further, it enters into cells, but, due to the absence of an OH group, cannot be further metabolized as normal glucose, fluorodeoxyglucose remaining in the cell until the complete decay of [18]F. For this reason

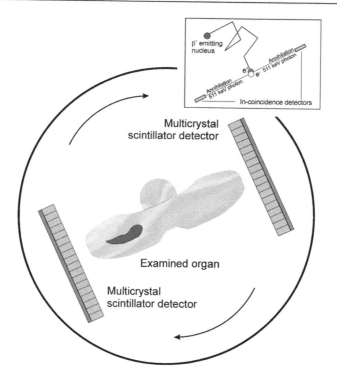

Figure 3.22 The reciprocal distribution of multicrystal detectors and examined body in the case of PET. The inset illustrates the multistage process of positron annihilation and the emission in the opposite direction of a couple of 511 keV photons. The positron emission and the annihilation are neither coincident in space nor in time.

Table 3.2 The Characteristic of the Main Radioisotopes Used in PET

Radioisotope	Positrons' Maximum Energy (MeV)	Half-Life (min)	Production
^{11}C	0.97	20.4	$^{14}N(p,\alpha)^{11}C$
^{13}N	1.19	9.97	$^{16}O(p,\alpha)^{13}N$
^{15}O	1.72	2.05	$^{14}N(d,n)^{15}O$
^{18}F	0.64	109.7	$^{18}O(p,n)^{18}F$

fluorodeoxyglucose is a good proxy for glucose metabolism, especially for high glucose-using cells such as cancer, kidney, brain, or brown adipocytes.

Including ^{18}F, the only disadvantage of the positron emission radioisotopes can be related to their short half-life time which implies the use of particle accelerators located as close as possible in the vicinity of radiodiagnostic centres. For this purpose, the dedicated cyclotrons or linear accelerators able to deliver the necessary current of protons and deuterons have been developed. In spite of these, the continuously extending number of PET installations proves that these inconveniences have in great measure been overcome.

PET belongs to the emissive computed tomographic techniques characterized by a low spatial resolution. This fact determines a certain uncertainty in the localization of the radiopharmaceutic-marked organ with respect to neighbouring anatomic structures as well as in representing its contour. This disadvantage can be overcome by combining it with CT whose resolution is of the order of magnitude of mm with PET.

The combined PET-CT examination allows a better correction for the annihilation photons in examined body, similar to the SPECT-CT case. With respect to SPECT the errors induced by photon self-absorption are about half as small taking into account that in the case of soft tissue, the LAC corresponding to ^{99m}Tc 140 keV gamma rays is about 1.9 times higher than in the case of 511 keV annihilation photons [8]. On the other hand, the PET correction for self-attenuation is independent of the source depth as the sum of the annihilation photon path depends only on the total body thickness along the photon path. This can be easily measured using lasers so the self-attenuation correction can be done with higher precision and accuracy.

All these advantages at present have made PET together with functional nuclear magnetic resonance imaging the most widely spread functional imaging techniques.

Dosimetry and Risk Associated with Nuclear Imaging

The high-energy ionizing radiation used in medical imaging, e.g., X- and gamma rays, transports a quantity of energy exceeding by a few orders of magnitude the binding energy of atoms which compose the organic molecules characteristic of any living organism. As mentioned before, when passing through matter, X- and gamma rays transfer their energy partially or totally to irradiated tissue by means of secondary electrons which, in turn, generate along their path multiple excitations and ionizations. This results in a multitude of free radicals, mainly consisting of neutral OH or charged OH$^-$ and H$^+$ radicals generated by the radiolysis of water molecules, radicals which are extremely reactive. As water represents the main component of cells, these radicals can interact with other components of living cells which can alter their function. Besides this, ionizing radiation can directly damage the DNA molecules by splitting one or both chains which could significantly impair its function. As DNA molecules control the entire cell activity, its damage can result in cell death or in its malignancy. For this reason the DNA is about 100 times more sensitive to the radiation than the rest of cell.

As the effects of radiation depend on the total amount of ionization and excitation, the quantity of absorbed energy depends on the absorption properties of the irradiated body and the amount of incident radiation and is characterized by the absorbed dose D defined as the quantity of energy absorbed by ionization per unit mass. In SI, the dose is expressed in grey (Gy), defined as one joule of energy absorbed per kilogram of matter [27].

According to the International Agency of Atomic Energy, ionizing radiation, depending on the absorbed dose, can produce in living individuals, including human ones, deterministic and stochastic effects.

The first category of effects, i.e., the deterministic ones, can occur if the absorbed dose exceeds a certain threshold, their severity, due to cell necrosis, being positively correlated with the absorbed dose. Below the threshold, these effects cannot be detected. Above the threshold, the deterministic effects are reproducible and, in a great measure, predictable. For instance, acute radiation syndromes, skin burns, cataracts, or tissue necrosis are considered deterministic effects. Being predictable and dose dependent, the deterministic effects such as tumours and necrosis are the basis of radiotherapy.

Opposite to deterministic effects, the stochastic which appear randomly at low absorbed doses can be associated with the development of cancer in tissue or organs exposed to radiation. The likelihood of stochastic effects occurring has no threshold but is proportional to the dose received. As a rule, stochastic effects occur after a latency of many years, their severity being independent of the initial received dose. In virtue of their stochastic character, it is possible only to predict the probability of developing a cancer.

In the case of a living organism, given the biological effectiveness of the radiation, i.e., the effectiveness of different types of radiation to generate the same biological effect, to characterize in an unitary matter different types of radiation by taking into account their effect on living matter, the absorbed dose D is replaced by the equivalent dose H. Accordingly, the equivalent dose defines the stochastic health effects of different types of ionizing radiation on the human body characterized by the probability of inducing genetic damage and cancer. Equivalent dose is thus defined for any type of ionizing radiation and its energy. In SI, the equivalent dose is expressed in sievert (Sv).

Equivalent dose is a dose quantity H representing the stochastic health effects, and it estimates the probability of radiation-induced cancer and genetic damage to appear after a single or multiple exposure to ionizing radiation. It is derived from the physical absorbed dose D, taking into account the biological effectiveness of the radiation, which is dependent on the radiation type and its energy. In the SI, the unit of measure is the sievert (Sv) expressed similar to absorbed dose, as the energy absorbed per kilogram of matter.

Accordingly, the equivalent dose H is defined as:

$$H = W_R D \qquad (3.24)$$

where W_R represents the radiation weighting factor whose value is defined by regulations and depends on the radiation energy and its type; D represents the absorbed dose.

In the case of X- and gamma rays the radiation weighting factor equals unit.

The third parameter which connects the absorbed dose to stochastic health effects is represented by the effective dose E. It is defined as the tissue-weighted sum of the equivalent dose for tissue exposed to radiation, each type of tissue being characterized by its weight factor W_T, regardless of whether the source of radiation is external or internal (Table 3.3). The

Table 3.3 The Numerical Values of the Tissue Weighting Factor According to [27]

Organ	W_T	Organ	W_T
Gonads	0.08	Liver	0.04
Red bone marrow	0.12	Oesophagus	0.04
Colon	0.12	Thyroid	0.04
Lung	0.12	Skin	0.01
Stomach	0.12	Bone surface	0.01
Breasts	0.12	Salivary glands	0.01
Bladder	0.04	Brain	0.01
Gross total			1.00

Table 3.4 The Effective Dose E for Different Types of Examination [28,29,30]

Examination	Target Organs	E (mSv)	Examination	Target Organs	E (mSv)
Radiography	Chest	0.1	CT	Head	2–4
	Extremities	0.001		Chest	7
	Spine	1.5		Heart	3–12
	Dental	0.005		Abdomen and pelvis	3–20
	Mammography	0.4		Colonography	6
	Lower extremity angiography	0.3–1.6		Gastrointestinal series	6–8
Densitometry	Bone density	0.001		Spine	6
PET + CT	Combined imaging	25	SPEC + CT	Combined imaging	11–15

Note: for comparison, the average annual natural background is 2.4 mSv [31] while in some EU countries, the maximum permitted annual dose for non-occupational public exposure is 1 mSv [32].

effective dose E is calculated by taking into account the contribution of each organ and tissue to the normal function of the whole organism. Unlike the absorbed dose, the effective dose as the equivalent one quantifies the stochastic health risk to the whole body when exposed to high-energy ionizing radiations. As mentioned before, this risk characterizes the probability of cancer induction and genetic effects in the case of low levels of ionizing radiation.

Derived from the equivalent dose, the effective dose E is expressed in sievert (Sv) too. It is worth mentioning that in both cases of H and E, connected to stochastic effects, 1 Sv represents a 5.5% chance of developing cancer [27]. In this regard it is worth mentioning that the effective dose is defined as a measure of stochastic effects, contrary to the absorbed dose which is intended as a measure of deterministic health effects.

All exposed medical imaging techniques use high-penetrating ionizing radiation, either X- or gamma rays, all of them transporting and releasing in tissue at the atomic level energy prone to generate highly reactive free radicals able to alter the vital processes of living cells.

For this reason, according to the ALARA principle, there should be a permanent balance between the gain of a correct diagnosis and the detriment produced by the harm caused by high ionizing radiation. As numerical values concerning the effective dose during different imaging investigations are of the order of magnitude of a few mSv (Table 3.4), it is obvious that all of these procedures are within the domain of stochastic effects. The general data reproduced in Table 3.4 show a certain degree of hierarchization, X-ray radiography being less harmful than CT which, in turn, is exceeded by PET-CT examinations. All of them should be regarded by taking into account that, according to existing regulations, and the EU are among the most restrictive, the annual limit for non-occupational public exposure of 1 mSv [04] is comparable with the effective dose received during a radiographic examination, but significantly lower in the case of CT and PET-CT examination. These particularities should always be taken into consideration when a certain type of medical imaging which implies the use of high-energy ionizing radiation must be prescribed.

Acknowledgement

Dedicated to Professor Vassileios Proimos.

References

1. Röntgen, W.C. (1986) Ueber eine neue Art von Strahlen, Sitzungsberichte der Würzburger Physik.-medic. *Gesellschaft*, Jg. 1–9. (In German) https://www.deutschestextarchiv.de/book/view/roentgen_strahlen02_1896?p=4 (accessed 19.03.2021).

2. Villard, P. (1900) Sur le rayonnement du radium. *C. R. Acad. Sci.* 130, 1178–9 (in French).

3. Sethi, A. (2006) X-rays: Interaction with matter, in: *Encyclopedia of medical devices and instrumentation*, (J.C. Webster, ed.), Wiley, 590–9.

4. Russo, P. ed. (2018) *Handbook of X-ray imaging, physics and technology*, Taylor & Francis, p. 1419.

5. Epstein, C.L. (2008) *Introduction to the mathematics of medical imaging*, Society for Industrial and Applied Mathematics, Philadelphia, PA, p. 793.

6. Uffmann, M., Schaefer-Prokop, C. (2009) Digital radiography: The balance between image quality and required radiation dose. *Eur J Radiol.* 72, 202–8.

7. Knoll, G. (2010) *Radiation detection and measurement,* Wiley, p. 830.

8. National Institute for Standard and Technology (2021) https://www.nist.gov/pml/x-ray-mass-attenuation-coefficients (accessed 10.05.2021)

9. Dance, D.R., Evans, S.H., Skinner, C.L., Bradley, A.G. (2012) Diagnostic radiology with X-rays, in: *Webb's Physics of Medical Imaging,* (M.A. Flower, ed.), CRC Press, pp. 13–95.

10. Sprawls, P. (1995) *Physical principles of medical imaging,* Medical Physics Publishing, Madison, p. 656.

11. Curry, T.S., Dowdey, J.E., Murry, R.C. (1990) *Christensen's physics of diagnostic radiology.* 4th ed., Williams & Wilkins, p. 535.

12. Hall, C., Lewis, R. (2019) Synchrotron radiation biomedical imaging and radiotherapy: From the UK to the Antipodes. *Phil. Trans. R. Soc. A* 377, 20180240.

13. Barrett, H.H., Swindell, W. (1981) *Radiological Imaging,* Academic Press, p. 693.

14. Boreman, G.D. (2021) *Modulation transfer function in optical and electro-optical systems,* SPIE Press, p. 140.

15. Kandel, E.R., Jessell, T.M., Schwartz, J.H., Siegelbaum, S.A., Hudspeth, A.J. (2013). *Principles of neural science.* 5th ed., McGraw-Hill, New York, p. 1709.

16. Gurney, R.W., Mott, N.F. (1938) The theory of photolysis of silver bromideand the photographic latent image. *Proc. R. Soc. London, Ser. A* 164, 151–167.

17. Lanconelli, N., Stefano Rivetti, S. (2015) *Review of detectors available for full-field digital mammography in: Radiation detectors for medical imaging* (J. Iwanczyk, ed.), CRC Press, Boca Raton, FL.

18. Herman, G.T. (2009) *The fundamentals of computerized tomography, Image reconstruction from projections,* 2nd ed., Springer, p. 293.

19. Radon, J. (1917) Über die Bestimmung von Funktionen durch ihre Integralwerte längs gewisser Mannigfaltigkeiten. *Berichte über die Verhandlungen der Königlich-Sächsischen Akademie der Wissenschaften zu Leipzig, Mathematisch-Physische Klasse,* 69, 262–277. (in German).

20. Schofield, R., King, L., Tayal, U., Castellano, I., Stirrup, J., Pontana, F., Earls, J., Nicol, E. (2020) Image reconstruction: Part 1 – Understanding filtered back projection, noise and image acquisition - Review article. *J. Cardiovasc. Comput. Tom.* 14, 219–225.

21. Webb, S. (2012) Mathematics of image formation and image processing, in: *Webb's Physics of Medical Imaging,* (M.A. Flower, ed.), CRC Press, pp. 687–711.

22. Ramachandran, G.N., Lakshminarayanan, A.V. (1971) Three-dimensional reconstruction from radiographs and electron micrographs: Application of convolutions instead of Fourier transforms. *Proc. Nat. Acad. Sci.* 68, 2236–2240.

23. Shepp, L.A., Logan, B.F. (1974) The Fourier reconstruction of a head section. *IEEE Trans. Nucl. Sci.* 21, 21–43.

24. Khalil, M.M. (2010) Elements of gamma camera and SPECT systems, in *Basic sciences of nuclear medicine,* (M.M. Khalil, ed.), Springer, pp. 155–178.

25. Chua,S., Groves, A. (2014) *Biomedical positron emission tomography (PET) imaging, in: Biomedical imaging. Applications and advances,* (P. Morris, ed.), Woodhead Publishing, Swaston, pp. 3–30.

26. Dietze, M.M.A., Branderhorst, W., Kunnen, B., Viergever, M.A., de Jong, H.W.M.A. (2019). Accelerated SPECT image reconstruction with FBP and an image enhancement convolutional neural network. *European Journal of Nuclear Medicine and Molecular Imaging Physics,* 6, 14–26

27. ICRP (2007). The 2007 recommendations of the international commission on radiological protection. *Annals of the ICRP,* 103, 62–77.

28. https://www.radiologyinfo.org/en/info.cfm?pg=safety-xray (Accessed 05.05.2021).

29. Brisbane, W., Bailey, M.R., Sorensen, M.D. (2016) An overview of kidney stone imaging techniques. *Nature Reviews Urology,* 13, 654–662.

30. Brindhaban, A. (2020) Effective dose to patients from SPECT and CT during myocardial perfusion imaging. *Journal of Nuclear Medicine Technology,* 48, 143–147.

31. United Nations Scientific Committee on the Effects of Atomic Radiation (2008). *Sources and effects of ionizing radiation, report to the general assembly with scientific annexes,* vol. II, United Nations, New York (published 2010).

32. Council Directive 2013/59/EURATOM of of 5 December 2013 laying down basic safety standards for protection against the dangers arising from exposure to ionising radiation, and repealing Directives 89/618/Euratom, 90/641/Euratom, 96/29/Euratom, 97/43/Euratom and 2003/122/Euratom, https://eur-lex.europa.eu/legal-content/EN/TXT/?uri=OJ:L:2014:013:TOC (accessed 04.06.2021).

4

Cone-Beam Computed Tomography Applications in Dentistry

Zühre Akarslan, Nursel Arpay, and Hatice Tetik

Introduction

Cone-beam computed tomography (CBCT) is an imaging technique providing three-dimensional assessment of the dental and maxillofacial region. The first introduction of a three-dimensional imaging system with cone-beam was in the 1970s. This made it easier to take a three-dimensional image in a shorter time. Subsequently, this technique was used for vascular imaging.

The first CBCT machine for dental use was introduced in 1998. This machine had a 15 × 15 cm cylinder reconstruction volume, 360° scan angle, 70 sec scan time, and worked at 110 kVp and 15 mA (maximum). The X-ray beam was pulsed, and the X-ray area detector was a special image intensifier coupled with a CCD TV camera. This system was capable of obtaining images in axial, coronal, sagittal, and cross-sectional planes. Also, a three-dimensional reconstruction of the area could be made.

With the advances in technology, CBCT has passed many milestones. Machines with simpler patient positioning, lower exposure time, different field of views (FOV), and better image qualities have been developed. Special exposure modes, such as children, adults, high-resolution, high definition, and endodontics, are also present with the improvement of the sensors.[1]

Before the CBCT machines were invented, CT was used for three-dimensional radiographic investigation of the oral and maxillofacial region. Reformatted two-dimensional images perpendicular to the jaws were achieved with special software in CT. This was especially used in the pre-operative assessment of the bone and anatomic structures in the implant site before implant surgery. However, CT has a higher cost, higher radiation dose, and lower spatial resolution compared to CBCT.[2,3] The main difference between the two techniques is the geometry of the X-rays passing through the patient. CT uses fan-beam X-ray geometry while CBCT uses cone-beam X-ray geometry. In the CBCT units the volume is generated from the reconstruction of the two-dimensional X-ray projections taken in a circular orbit around the patient.[4]

DOI: 10.1201/9781003112068-4

CBCT has some advantages and disadvantages compared to CT. The main differences between CBCT and CT are summarized in Table 4.1.[5]

Parts of the System, Image Acquisition, and Reconstruction

The main parts of the CBCT system are the X-ray tube, X-ray spectrum and imaging parameters, gantry, and detector. The X-rays are generated in an X-ray tube and directed to the area of interest with a collimator. Machines having different FOV sizes have a collimator with different pre-defined openings or freely adjustable collimation along the z-direction.

The gantry type differs among CBCT systems. Most of them have a fixed C-arm gantry usually rotating in the horizontal plane. This type of gantry is used in the systems in which patients sit or stand during the CBCT scan. C-arms or fixed gantries in which the tube and detector rotate in the vertical plane are used in systems in which patients lie back during the CBCT scan. The detectors convert X-ray photons to light photons which in turn are converted to electrical signals. In the early machines image intensifiers were commonly used as detectors, while different types of flat panel detectors are used in modern machines.

The X-ray tube and detector turn around the patient's head, and several two-dimensional images (raw data) are obtained during this period. Subsequently, these projections are reconstructed to form a three-dimensional image.[4,6] Some CBCT systems use pulsed and some use continuous X-ray exposure. In the majority of the systems, the tube and the detector make a full rotation around the patient while in some systems they make a half rotation. Besides, some systems give the opportunity to select a half or full rotation. Although the radiation dose decreases in half rotating systems, the overall image quality decreases also.

The aberrations associated with variations in detector dark current, gain, and pixel defects are removed in the pre-processing step before the reconstruction of the raw data. The scanned object is reconstructed as a three-dimensional matrix of voxels. Each voxel is assigned a grey value according to the X-ray attenuation of the scanned object. The scanned object's material composition is a determining factor of X-ray attenuation. This can be visualized in axial,

Table 4.1 Main Differences between CBCT and CT

	CBCT	CT
X-ray geometry	Conical or pyramidal	Fan-beam
Orthogonal image slices	Produced from the primary volumetric data	Produced from the axial slices obtained from the primary reconstruction of the data
Soft tissue visualization	Low	High
Radiation dose	Low	High
Cost	Cost-effective	Expensive
System operation	Easy	Difficult
Scatter radiation	High	Low
Image contrast	Low	High
Image noise	High	Low

sagittal, coronal, and cross-sectional planes and three-dimensional reconstructed volumes. This technique also allows multiple scans to be merged into one image. This procedure is called image stitching.

Correct patient positioning and a proper FOV area are important factors for obtaining an optimal image of the investigated area and minimizing the radiation exposure of the patient. In the CBCT technique the sectional image is obtained by the movement of the X-ray tube and film in opposite directions during an exposure. The object must be placed correctly in the focal plane to achieve an optimal image. Unwanted structures in the exposure path are blurred when they are not in the focal plane. CBCT machines use different patient positioning. Patients stand stationary in some machines, and sit or lie back in the others during X-ray exposure.[5]

The FOV dimension is an important factor for protecting potentially radiosensitive tissues from X-ray exposure during a CBCT scan. With the increase in the FOV dimensions a larger area will be irradiated. For example, the thyroid is a very radiosensitive tissue which will be directly in the exposure area. On the other hand, when we increase the width of the X-ray beam, the tissues in the exposure area will be irradiated with a higher radiation dose.[7]

Artefacts

Artefacts are unwanted images on radiographs caused by technical or processing errors. The recognition of artefacts is important for the proper diagnosis of pathology. Similar to other imaging techniques, artefacts could occur in the CBCT technique. The reason for artefacts in CBCT is the discrepancy between the mathematical modelling used for three-dimensional reconstruction and the actual physical conditions. Beam-hardening, extinction, partial volume effect, aliasing, and ring and motion artefacts are among the reported artefacts in CBCT imaging. Generally, the most seen artefact is beam hardening.[4] Metal artefacts are common on CBCT images as metal-containing materials are commonly used in restorative and prosthetic treatment. Prosthetic treatment of a missing tooth with an implant, orthodontic treatment with metallic braces, metal-containing crowns, and amalgam restorations of decayed teeth are common treatment modalities in dentistry. Therefore, during a CBCT scan, these dense objects absorb a high amount of X-rays and lead to artefacts. These dense materials can cause beam hardening, resulting in cupping artefacts, and dark bands and streaks on the image. The motion artefact is the other common artefact on CBCT images. It happens when the patient moves during the X-ray exposure. It is seen as parallel lines to the movement direction on the image.

Different methods are used to reduce the artefacts in CBCT imaging. In the past, these were generally about post-processing algorithms operating on the three-dimensional volume dataset obtained from the scan of the object.[8,9] Nowadays, with the use of artificial intelligence learning models in radiology, a convolutional neural network was successful in reducing screw artefacts.[10–13]

Examples of beam hardening and motion artefacts are given in Figures 4.1 and 4.2.

The Use of CBCT in Dentistry

CBCT is generally used in oral and maxillofacial surgery, orthodontics, periodontology, endodontics, and pedodontics. Implant planning, radiographic investigation of third molars, impacted teeth, temporomandibular joint, odontogenic cysts and tumours, trauma,

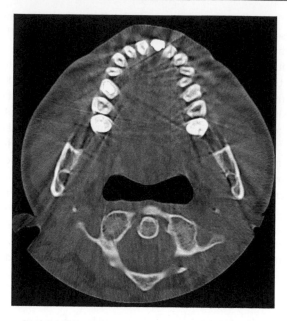

Figure 4.1 Beam hardening in CBCT.

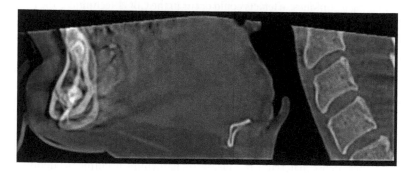

Figure 4.2 Motion artefact in CBCT.

osteomyelitis, bisphosphonate-related osteonecrosis of the jaws, mini-implant placement in orthodontics, sinus pathologies, cleft lip and palate, tooth and jaw fractures, and orthognathic surgery were reported among the common indications of CBCT.[14,15]

Oral and Maxillofacial Surgery

CBCT is an important advanced imaging technique in oral and maxillofacial surgery. Three-dimensional evaluation with multiplanar views helps the surgeon in diagnosis, pre-operative treatment planning, and post-operative evaluation when two-dimensional radiography does not provide adequate information. Images are obtained without any distortion, magnification, or superimposition. However, detailed soft tissue imaging is inferior compared to CT. Thus, the soft tissue imaging of lesions, TMJ disc, and head and neck infections is not possible with this technique.

CBCT could be used in the following cases in oral and maxillofacial surgery:

- Implant planning: it provides volumetric assessment of the jaws with a lower radiation dose and cost compared to CT. CBCT is used for the identification of important anatomical relationships, bone morphology, bone volume and quality, augmentation procedures, grafting, distraction, zygoma implants, and evaluation of neighbouring teeth[16] (Figure 4.3).
- Treatment plan of a third molar tooth: the third molars are among the teeth having the highest impaction rate. An ideal radiographic examination should give information about the position of the tooth, the morphology, the number and development of the roots, the surrounding alveolar bone, and related anatomical structures. The most important factor is the relation of the mandibular third molars to the mandibular canal and the maxillary third molars to the sinus. The CBCT provides a clear assessment of the third molars with these anatomical structures.[17,18] The mandibular canal is especially important as it contains the inferior alveolar nerve. Any damage to this canal may result in nerve damage. In some cases, a two-dimensional panoramic image may be useful for radiographic evaluation; however, CBCT may be indicated if it is believed that it will change the treatment or the treatment outcome for the patient when there is a suspicion of a close contact between the tooth and the mandibular canal in the panoramic radiograph.[18]
  - Supernumerary teeth.
  - Bony components of the temporomandibular joint.
  - Jaw lesions: odontogenic cysts and tumours, osteomyelitis, bisphosphonate-related osteonecrosis of the jaws and other lesions.

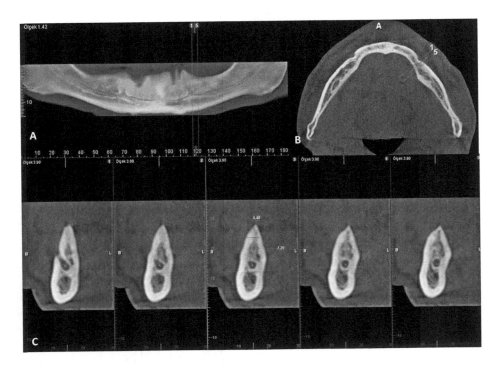

Figure 4.3 Implant planning.

- Orthognathic surgery.
- Sinus pathologies (oroantral fistula, etc.).
- Tooth and jaw fractures.

Examples of CBCT images in oral and maxillofacial surgery are given in Figures 4.3–4.8.

Orthodontics

Radiographic imaging is an important step in the diagnosis of orthodontic pathology and treatment outcomes of the patient. Generally two-dimensional radiography is adequate for these purposes. However, these techniques present some limitations, and patients may require three-dimensional imaging in complex cases.

CBCT could be used in the following cases in orthodontics:

- Impacted canine teeth: this is probably the most common indication for CBCT investigation in orthodontics. The correct location of the tooth, the relationship of the impacted tooth with adjacent teeth and important anatomic structures, evaluation of the dental follicle, associated pathologies, and teeth resorption could be assessed with CBCT. It provides superior radiographic examination of impacted teeth compared to two-dimensional techniques as superimposition doesn't occur in CBCT. CBCT is useful in surgical procedures as the accurate location of the crown of the tooth can be found.
- Assessment of root angulation, root morphology, and resorption.
- Quantity and quality of bone and anatomical structures in temporary anchorage device placement.
- Cleft lip and palate defects and outcomes of alveolar bone grafts.
- Temporomandibular joint morphology and pathology.
- Airway morphology and obstructive sleep apnoea.

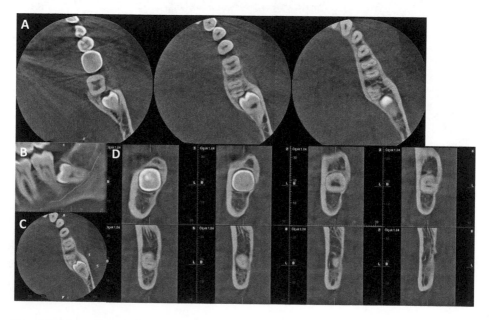

Figure 4.4 Impacted mandibular third molar.

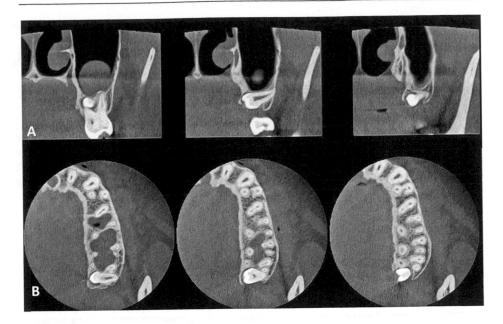

Figure 4.5 Supernumerary tooth.

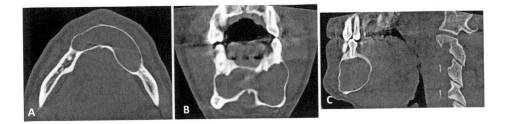

Figure 4.6 Large lesion in the mandible.

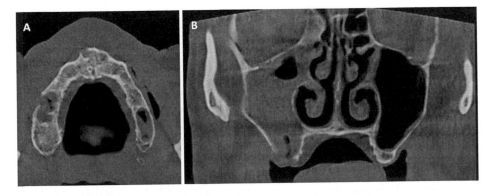

Figure 4.7 Oroantral fistula.

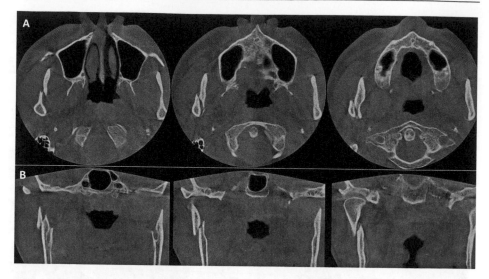

Figure 4.8 Fracture of the mandible.

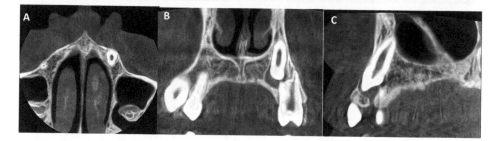

Figure 4.9 Impacted canine.

- Vertical malocclusion.
- Maxillary transverse dimension and maxillary expansion.[19]

Examples of CBCT images in orthodontics are given in Figures 4.9–4.11.

Periodontology

Radiographic investigation of the alveolar bone is a routine procedure in periodontology. It is usually made with two-dimensional intra-oral and extra-oral radiographic techniques. CBCT has high accuracy in the visualization of the supporting alveolar bone of the teeth in the bucco-lingual direction, vertical defects, and furcation involvement compared to two-dimensional techniques. Due to these advantages, practitioners have started to use CBCT especially in pre-operative diagnosis and surgical procedures in periodontology. This technique is useful in regenerative periodontal surgery of maxillary molars.

CBCT could be used in the following cases in periodontology:

- A CBCT scan should only be made in cases when the radiographic information obtained from two-dimensional imaging is insufficient. It should be only applied to complex periodontal cases particularly those involving the maxillary molars.[20]

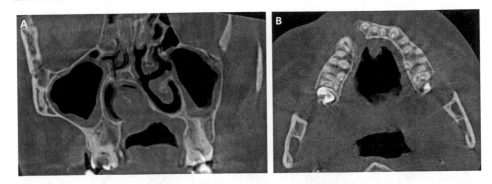

Figure 4.10 Cleft lip and palate.

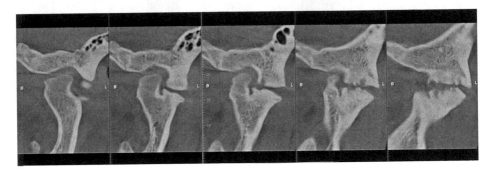

Figure 4.11 Ankilosis in the temporomandibular joint.

Examples of CBCT images in periodontology are given in Figures 4.12 and 4.13.

Endodontics

Radiological examination is important for diagnosis, treatment, and follow-up of treatment results in endodontics. High resolution and detail are required for clear monitoring of the root canal and surrounding periodontal tissues in CBCT. However, increasing resolution leads to an increase in radiation dose. To obtain high-resolution images with lower radiation doses, small FOV areas could be used, as small FOV dimensions reduce radiation exposure and scattering.[21]

CBCT could be used in the following cases in endodontics:

- Dental trauma and periapical pathology when periapical radiographs are insufficient: correct evaluation of the location and size of the pathology is important for the diagnosis, treatment, and follow-up process of periapical lesions. Periapical radiographs may not be sufficient to visualize small periapical lesions. This situation affects the decision between conservative treatment and endodontic treatment. The standard radiographic method used for the radiological detection of apical periodontitis is periapical radiography. However, it has disadvantages such as causing anatomical noise and inadequate early diagnosis.[22,23]
- Internal and external root resorption: correct diagnosis of internal and external root resorption in two-dimensional radiography is lower than with CBCT.[24]

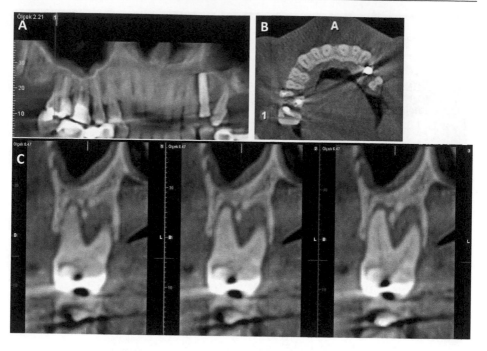

Figure 4.12 Alveolar bone destruction of a maxillary molar tooth.

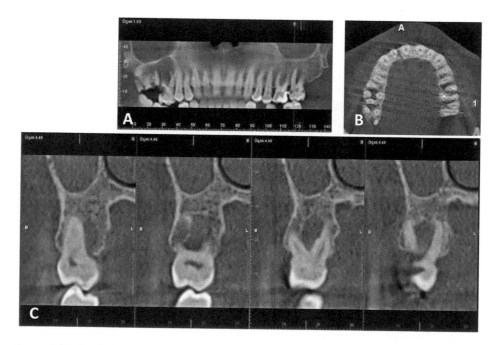

Figure 4.13 Alveolar bone destruction in the furcation of a maxillary tooth.

- Accessory root canals: accessory root canals that cannot be detected as a result of clinical and radiological examination may adversely affect the prognosis of endodontic treatment. To prevent such situations, the use of CBCT gives good results.[25-27]
- C-shaped root canals: C-shaped canals are anatomical variations that can develop as a result of root fusion, often observed in the second molar teeth in the mandible. It has been stated that it may be appropriate to use CBCT pre-operatively to avoid the difficulties that may arise in the localization, cleaning, and shaping of the root canal system.[22]
- Dens evaginatus: dens evaginatus occurs when the inner enamel epithelium and the ectomesenchymal cells of the dental papilla proliferate and fold in an extraordinary manner into the stellate reticulum of the enamel organ, which is thought to develop in the bell stage of tooth development. It appears as a cusp-like elevation of enamel, referred to as a tubercle.[28] Type III dens evaginatus extending to the root is especially clinically important. The use of CBCT is recommended for the diagnosis and treatment of this type.[22]
- Palatogingival grooves: the palatogingival groove is the developmental groove in the root, usually found in the palatal region of the maxillary incisors.[29]

    It is a rare developmental dental anomaly that can cause periodontal pocket, bone destruction, and pulp necrosis in teeth. Periapical radiographs may be incomplete developmental abnormalities in imaging because they provide two-dimensional images. In these cases, the use of CBCT will be very useful for early diagnosis and treatment.[22]
- Assessment of the outcome of root canal treatment: studies have shown that the success of canal treatments evaluated by periapical radiography is lower than the success of treatments evaluated with CBCT. It was seen that root canal fillings made by evaluating with CBCT were of lower quality than the treatments performed by evaluating with periapical radiography.[23]

Examples of CBCT images in endodontics are given in Figures 4.14 and 4.15.

Pedodontics

The use of CBCT in pedodontics is more limited compared to adults. The exposure time of a CBCT scan differs according to many factors, but it is generally higher than two-dimensional radiographic techniques. This makes the cooperation of the child harder and may lead to motion artefacts as the child has a higher likelihood to move during the X-ray exposure. This should be kept in mind when the child lacks adequate cooperation for dental procedures.

The thyroid gland, breast tissue, and gonads of the children are more sensitive to radiation compared to adults. The cancer risk per Sievert of children is higher than in adults.[30] With the global acceptance of the CBCT technique, more CBCT scans have started to be used with children. The risk-benefit ratio of CBCT examinations in children should be made more carefully in each case.[1]

A CBCT may be indicated in the following cases in pedodontics:

- When the source of an acute dental or bone infection could not be found with two-dimensional radiographic techniques.
- Trauma cases with a suspicion of root fractures.
- Cleft lip and palate cases to determine the boundaries and location of the cleft.

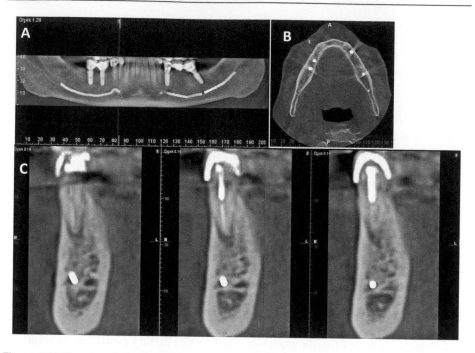

Figure 4.14 Chronic apical periodontitis in a mandibular premolar.

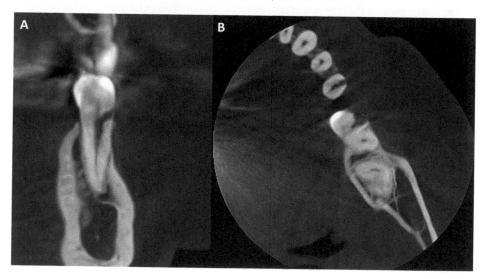

Figure 4.15 A resorption cavity in a mandibular premolar.

- Dental resorption cases when two-dimensional radiography does not reveal enough information.
- Large cysts, tumours, and other bone pathologies to show the accurate boundaries of the lesions and its relationship with the neighbouring anatomical structures.[31]

The worldwide acceptance of CBCT has raised several concerns about unnecessary use of the system due to harmful effects of radiation. Therefore, it is important to understand the

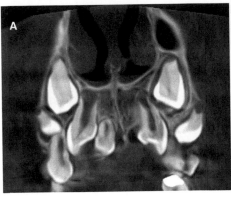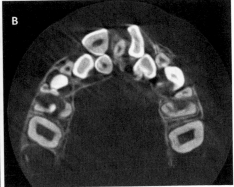

Figure 4.16 A supernumerary tooth in a child.

technical properties and indications to minimize radiation risk to the patient, radiology department staff, and environment.[6] At this point, the "as low as reasonably achievable" (ALARA) principle was suggested to be modified to the "as low as diagnostically acceptable" (ALADA) principle. An appropriate indication, proper FOV dimensions, adjustment of mA, kVp, and selection of high definition/high resolution of the scanning protocol should be made to obtain images according to the ALADA principle.[1,6]

Examples of CBCT images in pedodontics are given in Figure 4.16.

Conclusion

CBCT has an important role in three-dimensional imaging in dentistry. It continues to gain popularity in many dental applications. However, practitioners should be aware of the possible risks of radiation exposure and use this technique according to the ALADA principle. CBCT scans should be made when they add radiographic information or change the treatment modality.

References

1. Jaju PP, Jaju SP. Cone-beam computed tomography: Time to move from ALARA to ALADA. *Imaging Sci Dent.* 2015;45:263–5.

2. Ames JR, Johnson RP, Stevens EA. Computerized tomography in oral and maxillofacial surgery. *J Oral Surg.* 1980;38:145.

3. Mozzo P, Procacci C, Tacconi A, et al. A new volumetric CT machine for dental imaging based on the cone-beam technique: Preliminary results. *Eur Radiol.* 1998;8(9):1558–64.

4. Schulze R, Heil U, Grob D, et al. Artefacts in CBCT: A review. *Dentomaxillofac Radiol.* 2011;40:265–73.

5. Scarfe WC, Li Z, Aboelmaaty W, et al. Maxillofacial cone beam computed tomography: Essence, elements and steps to interpretation. *Aust Dent J.* 2012;57(1 Suppl):46–60.

6. Pauwels R, Araki K, Siewerdsen JH, et al. Technical aspects of dental CBCT: State of the art. *Dentomaxillofac Radiol*. 2015;44:20140224.

7. Ludlow JB, Timothy R, Walker C, et al. Effective dose of dental CBCT-a meta analysis of published data and additional data for nine CBCT units. *Dentomaxillofac Radiol*. 2014;44:20140197.

8. Altunbas MC, Shaw CC, Chen L, et al. A post-reconstruction method to correct cupping artefacts in cone beam breast computed tomography. *Med Phys*. 2007;34:3109–18.

9. Tuy HK. A post-processing algorithm to reduce metallic clip artefacts in CT images. *Eur Radiol*. 1993;3:129–34.

10. Thies M, Zäch JN, Gao C, et al. A learning-based method for online adjustment of C-arm cone-beam CT source trajectories for artifact avoidance. *Int J Comput Assist Radiol Surg*. 2020;15(11):1787–96.

11. Ketcha MD, Marrama M, Souza A, et al. Sinogram + image domain neural network approach for metal artifact reduction in low-dose cone-beam computed tomography. *J Med Imaging (Bellingham)*. 2021;8(5):052103.

12. Lee D, Park C, Lim Y, et al. Metal artifact reduction method using a fully convolutional network in the sinogram and image domains for dental computed tomography. *J Digit Imaging*. 2020;33(2):538–46.

13. Minnema J, van Eijnatten M, Hendriksen AA, et al. Segmentation of dental cone-beam CT scans affected by metal artifacts using a mixed-scale dense convolutional neural network. *Med Phys*. 2019;46(11):5027–35.

14. De Vos W, Casselman J, Swennen GR. Cone-beam computerized tomography (CBCT) imaging of the oral and maxillofacial region: A systematic review of the literature. *Int J Oral Maxillofac Surg*. 2009;38:609–25.

15. Akarslan Z, Peker İ. Bir diş hekimliği fakültesindeki konik ışınlı bilgisayarlı tomografi incelemesi istenme nedenleri. *Acta Odontol Turc*. 2015;32(1):1–6.

16. Jacobs R, Salmon B, Codari M, et al. Cone beam computed tomography in implant dentistry: Recommendations for clinical use. *BMC Oral Health*. 2018;18:88.

17. Yun-Hoa J, Bong-Hae C. Assessment of maxillary third molars with panoramic radiography and cone-beam computed tomography. *Imaging Sci Dent*. 2015;45(4):233–40.

18. Matzen LH, Wenzel A. Efficacy of CBCT for assessment of impacted mandibular third molars: A review – based on a hierarchical model of evidence. *Dentomaxillofac Radiol*. 2015;44:20140189.

19. Kapila SD, Nervina JM. CBCT in orthodontics: Assessment of treatment outcomes and indications for its use. *Dentomaxillofac Radiol*. 2015;44:20140282.

20. Woelber JP, Fleiner J, Rau J, et al. Accuracy and usefulness of CBCT in periodontology: A systematic review of the literature. *Int J Periodontics Restorative Dent*. 2018;38(2):289–97.

21. Lo Giudice R, Nicita F, Puleio F, et al. Accuracy of periapical radiography and CBCT in endodontic evaluation. *Int J Dent*. 2018;201(16):2514243.

22. Ertaş E, Arslan H, Çapar İ, et al. Endodontide konik ışınlı bilgisayarlı tomografi. *Atatürk Üniv Diş Hek Fak Derg.* 2014;24(1):113–8.

23. Patel S, Brown J, Pimentel T, et al. Cone beam computed tomography in endodontics–A review of the literature. *Int Endod J.* 2019;52(8):1138–52.

24. Estevez R, Aranguren J, Escorial A, et al. Invasive cervical resorption Class III in a maxillary central incisor: Diagnosis and follow-up by means of cone-beam computed tomography. *J Endod.* 2010;36:2012–4.

25. Kottoor J, Velmurugan N, Ballal S, et al. Four- rooted maxillary first molar having C-shaped palatal root canal morphology evaluated using cone-beam computerized tomography: A case report. *Oral Surg Oral Med Oral Pathol Oral Radiol Endod.* 2011;111:41–5.

26. Ayranci LB, Arslan H, Topcuoglu HS. Maxillary first molar with three canal orifices in mesio buccal root. *J Conserv Dent.* 2011;14:436–7.

27. Abella F, Mercade M, Duran-Sindreu F, et al. Managing severe curvature of radix entomolaris: Three-dimensional analysis with cone beam computed tomography. *Int Endod J.* 2011;44:876–85.

28. Chen JW, Huang GJ, Bakland LK. Dens evaginatus: Current treatment options. *JADA.* 2020;151(5):358–67.

29. Cho YD, Lee JE, Chung Y, et al. Collaborative management of combined periodontal-endodontic lesions with a palatogingival groove: A case series. *J Endod.* 2017;43(2):332–7.

30. Choi E, Ford NL. Measuring absorbed dose for i-CAT CBCTexaminations in child, adolescent and adult phantoms. *Dentomaxillofac Radiol.* 2015;44:20150018.

31. Horner K, Barry S, Dave M, et al. Diagnostic efficacy of cone beam computed tomography in paediatric dentistry: A systematic review. *Eur Arch Paediatr Dent.* 2020;21(4):407–26.

5

Role of Nanoparticles in Medical Imaging

Pratyusha Nayak, Reetuparna Nanda, and Monalisa Mishra

Introduction

In the 21st century, our understanding regarding physiological systems and the mechanism of manifestation of several diseases has improved significantly. The molecular mechanisms of several diseases have been decoded and used for treatment purposes. Advancements in biomedical technologies allow us to use them for diagnosis and healing purposes. These techniques involve less invasive or completely non-invasive methods for the detection of disease. Some biomedical techniques are used such as Magnetic Resonance Imaging (MRI) and Computed Tomography (CT) for the non-invasive imaging of disease and have reduced side effects as related to the conventional methods of radiography [1]. Imaging techniques like positron emission tomography (PET), ultrasonography, optical imaging, photo acoustic imaging, and single-photon emission computed tomography (SPECT) have also been developed and employed for the diagnosis of disease [2]. Along with the sophisticated techniques, several micro- and nanoparticles (NPs) from a wide variety of materials, like diverse kinds of biomolecules (protein, lipids) or metals like iron oxide, and materials like silica, carbon nanotubes, fullerenes, and microtubules, have been designed and employed for biomedical applications.

The size of NPs developed for imaging varies from 1 nm to <1 μm. The microparticles designed for imaging range from 1 μm to 1 mm. The diversity in size, types, characteristics, and properties allows them to be used in modern medical applications. Each nanomaterial has its unique physical, optical, and chemical properties for a specific application. NPs are used in the biomedical field for both diagnostic and treatment purposes. They provide information regarding the target molecule or tissue, to check the vascular permeability, to carry the drug to a targeted area, to release it, and to monitor the response after the release of the drug.

DOI: 10.1201/9781003112068-5

Henceforth, NP synthesis, characterization, and application are carried out extensively [3–6]. The NPs are fine-tuned to alter the absorption and emission properties for specific uses. NPs are either under trial or used for current clinical therapeutic and diagnostic purposes.

With the wide use of NPs, toxic reports are also coming from animal studies [7–10]. Thus, the physical as well as chemical properties of the NPs like shape, size, toxicity, hydrophilicity, and charge are taken into consideration before they are used for clinical studies. For instance, positively charged NPs are being used for increasing the phagocytosis process for cell labelling purposes [11]. The NPs like liposomes, micelles, solid lipid NPs, nanotubes, quantum dots, metallic NPs (gold, silver, iron oxide, etc.), dendrimers, and polymeric NPs are used for imaging applications. The current chapter summarizes different kinds of NPs that are in the trial phase for biomedical imaging, both *in vitro* and *in vivo*.

Nanoparticles Used in Biomedical Imaging

Many NPs have been used in recent times for biomedical imaging for the diagnosis of different types of diseases. Broadly they are categorized as (a) metallic NPs and (b) miscellaneous NPs. (a) The metallic NPs include gold NPs, iron oxide NPs, quantum dots, and carbon nanotubes. (b) The miscellaneous NPs include calcium phosphate NPs, perfluorocarbon NPs, lipid-based NPs, and polyelectrolyte complex NPs.

Metallic NPs for Imaging

Gold Nanoparticles

Many inorganic NPs including gold have great potential to be used for biomedical imaging because of their appropriate chemical, optical, and physical properties [12]. The properties that make gold NPs efficient for imaging include (a) awesome biocompatibility, (b) relatively less or negligible toxicity, (c) a high X-ray absorption coefficient, and (d) a heavy nucleus [13]. The gold NPs are manufactured from gold salt as the raw material (e.g., $AuCl4^-$), and the reducing agents used are trisodium citrate or sodium borohydride [14–16]. The gold NPs are used for computed tomography, colorimetric biosensing, and fluorescence resonance energy transfer (FRET).

Gold Nanoparticles in Computed Tomography (CT)

X-ray computed tomography (CT) is used to enhance the contrast between parts with different densities like the soft tissue and the electron-dense bone. Thus it is used for cancer diagnosis by using contrasting agents which are soluble in water and are small organic iodinated molecules. One of the major limitations of using these traditional contrasting agents in CT is that they have very short imaging times and are subject to frequent renal clearance [17–19]. To overcome this difficulty many gold NPs are introduced for contrast enhancement in X-ray CT. Gum Arabic stabilized gold NPs are biocompatible and also have very little plasma binding which ensures *in-vivo* stability [20]. PEG-coated gold NPs with anti-biofouling properties can extend the half-life in systemic circulation [21]. They are found in blood for more than four hours when injected into rats. This time duration is much higher than the time of any other contrasting agents. PEG-coated NPs enhance the contrast between hepatoma and normal tissue in the diseased rats during X-ray CT. The gold nanorods are used for detecting head and neck cancer using clinical computed tomography [22]. The gold nanorods along with UM-A9 antibodies are used for the detection of squamous cell carcinoma [23].

Thrombus-targeted gold NPs were used to detect blood clotting in mice. Using these NPs clots were visible in CT imaging 5 mins after injection in the mice and for the next three weeks. A tissue plasminogen activator was used to induce the breakdown of the clots; it consequently decreased the CT signals [24]. Gold NPs with a coating of linospiril is found to target ACE *in vivo*. This can be used to detect defects in the hearts and lungs. The NPs present in thiotic acid are stable and provide a good contrast *in vivo*, and free linospiril helps to scan at a low signal, thus confirming direct targeting [25].

Although bone does not require any contrasting agent for X-ray CT, to visualize micro damage or tissue implants gold NPs were proven to be appropriate. To target the NPs towards the bone, gold NPs were conjugated with glutamic acid so they can be attached to the bone as they chelate the calcium ions at the surface of the bone [26]. Gold NPs targeting kidney renal imaging techniques have been proven to be beneficial to diagnose different diseases including cancer. Less than 2 nm gold NPs coated with bovine serum albumin (BSA) were used for the diagnosis of kidney diseases. These NPs were compared with iopromide *in vivo* and *in vitro*. Similarly, CT attenuations were achieved with comparison to iopromide, and the renal imaging was high in resolution using a CT scan after 2 hours of the injection [27].

Gold NPs have the potential to be used in colorimetric assays [28]. The colours are changed by a change in plasmon resonance frequency which is dependent on the average distance between the gold NPs. As the process of agglomeration takes place, there is a chance that the colour might alter from red to purple or blue. With dispersion the colour change is seen in reverse order, i.e., from purple to red [29, 30]. This technique has recently been used in the detection of biomolecules like peptides, lipids, nucleic acid, or small molecules like metals (mercury) [31–33].

Use of Gold Nanoparticles for Fluorescence Resonance Energy Transfer (FRET)

Gold NPs are also used in FRET. They are being developed for the detection of DNA. This can be beneficial for the pathology, genetics, drug industry, pathogen detection, and clinical diagnosis of various diseases. Gold NP is also used for the identification of DNA cleavage, and this can help in the recognition of aberrant gene expression, increased mutation rates and the progression of cancer, and alterations in DNA sequence [34, 35]. This technique is mostly centred on either FRET or non-FRET-quenching mechanisms. There is an enhancement of signal observed after the cleavage of the DNA. But the FRET-based method has a limitation of the dipole-dipole mechanism which has a size constraint of less than 100 angstrom [36].

Iron Oxide NP

Iron is used to synthesize superparamagnetic iron oxide nanoparticles (SPIONs) having particle diameters greater than 50 nm. Ultra-small superparamagnetic iron oxide (USPIO) with diameters of less than 50 nm is used for the labelling of cells and stem cell imaging directly [37]. Its clinical application and pharmacokinetics can be modified by altering its size and surface coating [38]. These NPs have high magnetic moments and thus are capable of generating homogenous microscopic fields. They accumulate in particular organs and show a strong decrease in intensity [37]. When tissues were loaded with SPIONs the magnetic field helped to improve contrast in MRI. They are now more preferred in imaging techniques as they are better and safer than radioactive tracers. We describe the details of SPIO and USPIO nanoparticles in the MPS imaging section.

Quantum Dots

Quantum dots (QDs) are NPs with unique size and shape; they are semiconductors in nature and are widely used in medical diagnostics due to their distinctive electronic and optical properties. They are used in medicine bioimaging, diagnostics, single-molecule probes, and drug delivery. The optical features of the QDs can be altered by altering their size and composition. These properties make them an excellent candidate for *in-vivo* imaging to be resistant to photo-bleaching, high brightness, multiplexing capacity, and therapeutic delivery [39]. The synthesis of QDs mainly uses two different approaches: (a) the top-down method and (b) the bottom-up method. In the first method lithography [40] is used to obtain the QDs, while in the latter one the self-assembly of precursor materials takes place within the solution to give rise to the QDs.

QDs have advantages like (a) broad excitation spectra, (b) narrow emission spectra, and (c) huge Stokes shifts as compared to common organic dyes and luminescent proteins, (d) they are one hundred times brighter than normal dyes, and (e) they are very stable to photo-bleaching unlike the organic dyes [41, 42]. QDs show a florescence range from near ultraviolet to near-infrared (NIR). This is advantageous for biomedical applications because of the lesser auto-florescence and lower absorption by the tissues [42, 43]. QDs vary a lot in size when injected into the patient's body and and then the patient's body is exposed to a single wavelength which excites the QDs with minimal cross-talk and negligible overlap [44–46].

QDs have also been used in FRET immunoassays as biosensors and show better results than conventionally used organic dyes. The fluorescence spectra can be adjusted which allows good energy transfer and results in high quantum yields which makes the energy transfer very efficient. QDs have a symmetric and narrow-ranged emission spectrum which makes them easy to differentiate from the acceptor spectrum [47–50]. Though Quantum Dots have proven to have many biomedical applications, when they are entered into an in vivo system their properties, like aqueous solubility, stability, and toxicity, need further investigation.

Surface Modifications for Improved Efficiency

As well as having many applications for biomedical purposes QDs also face some major challenges at present such as insolubility in water. To tackle this problem, QDs are encapsulated inside hydrophilic materials like hydrogels. Surface capping and ligand exchange are the effective methods to improve the water solubility of QDs. The surface modification depends on the application of the QDs in *in vivo* environmental conditions [40]. Bioconjugated antibodies, small proteins, oligonucleotides, and small molecule ligands are bonded to the surface of the QDs for efficient use *in vitro* as well as *in vivo* [41, 51].

Carbon Nanotubes

Carbon nanotubes are excellent NPs due to their high surface area, thermal and electrical conductivity, and good mechanical strength [52–54]. Structurally there are two major types of carbon nanotubes: (a) single-walled (SWNT) and (b) multiple-walled (MWNT). Carbon nanotubes are used as biosensors because of their rich electronic properties [55, 56]. The nanotubes absorb EM waves in the near-infrared region due to which they have been used in heating cancer therapy [57]. SWNT is used for cellular and subcellular imaging [58–60]. It is available in two different types: one type uses intrinsic fluorescence, which includes the band-gap emission of semiconducting SWNTs which falls in near-IR as well as a visible range [61]. In the second type, a nanotube is attached to fluorescent or radioactive agents [62]. All the different types of SWNTs have band-gap fluorescence properties [62]. These carbon nanotubes do not undergo any chemical damage when the fluorescence emission is observed in the near-infrared region. The semiconducting SWNTs' diameter ranges from one nanometre to several hundred nanometres with emission ranges of 900–1,600 nm. The nanotube spectra are detected in complex biological environments because most biomolecules do not show any colours and nanotubes have a sharp spectrum. In some cases the band-gap fluorescence emission is delicate towards the surface of nanotubes. SWNTs and MWNTs with a defective outward region show comparatively robust photoluminescence after chemical functionalization at the defective sites, and with better functionalization better emission is detected [63]. The semiconducting SWNTs are used for probing cell surface receptors as near-IR fluorescent tags [64]. In this experiment carbon nanotubes were dispersed with a surfactant PL-PEG-NH2 which had terminal amine. This resulted in carbon nanotubes with amine groups, and then they were conjugated with thiolated Rituxan (an antibody recognizing CD20 cell surface receptor) and Herceptin (antibody recognizes the HER2/neu receptors present in some breast cancer cells). These improvised carbon nanotubes with conjugated antibodies when present in solution phase can give a spectral emission of 1,000–1,600 nm and excitation at 785 nm. Pluronic surfactant-dispersed pristine SWNTs were investigated to check the uptake of macrophage-like cells and used near-IR fluorescence [58]. For this, the macrophage samples were dispersed in the media which already have SWNTs with attached surfactants. Later, the fluorescence intensity was measured for some time which showed a smooth increase. The localizations of nanotubes were detected in the intracellular vesicles. Although carbon nanotubes mostly included florescence-based imaging, some other imaging techniques like radioisotope tracing and microscopy techniques were also used for some *in vitro* and *in vivo* analysis [60, 65, 66]. SWNTs were detected inside the cells through low-loss energy-filtered transmission electron microscopy in amalgamation with electron energy loss spectrum [67]. This technique allows the visualization of the stained as well as unstained cells.

Dendrimers

Dendrimers are the most frequently researched polymers. The first dendrimer family was described in a research paper about polyamidoamine (PAMAM) dendrimers [68, 69]. This dendrimer is properly characterized and the best-understood series in the modern era [70]. A dendrimer is globular in shape having (a) a core, (b) an interior of shells, and (c) the terminal functional groups [70]. In the spherical shape, there are a lot of branching points which show characteristics like monodispersity and nanometric size range. Their structure gives them the flexibility to adjust the solubility, molecular dimension, polarity, density, size, shape, and flexibility. The selection of the terminal functional groups affects the physical and chemical properties of the nanostructure. Their shape is beneficial for easy penetration into the cell and the lipophilic surface [71]. Henceforth, they are used as a mode of transportation for transporting the drug, antibodies, and hormones.

Communications between Drug Molecules and Dendrimers

A dendrimer interacts with drug molecules both physically and chemically. Physical interaction involves non-bonding interactions amongst precise groups between the dendrimer and the drug which leads to simple encapsulation. This is also favoured due to the spherical shape of the dendrimer with empty cavities which enables the interaction of less soluble drugs which have hydrophobic interactions [72–74]. The dendrimer can chemically interact with drugs in two possible ways; the first is electrostatic interactions while the second one is the conjugation of any drug to the dendrimer. Functional groups like amine and carboxylic acid boost the solubility of hydrophobic drugs as they are present in high quantities on the surface of the dendrimers [75]. Non-steroidal anti-inflammatory drugs (NSAIDs) with carboxyl groups like ibuprofen [76], indomethacin [77], and piroxicam [77] form electrostatic interactions thus resulting in a stable complex [78]. Active moeties like PEG and p-amino benzoic acid along with biodegradable linkages like amides and ester bonds are covalently conjugated to dendrimers to form a "prodrug". Examples of drugs that get conjugated with PAMAM dendrimers are naproxen [79], penicillin V [80], and propranolol [81].

Use of Dendrimers in Magnetic Resonance Imaging (MRI)

Dendrimers are applied as contrast agents for macromolecular MRI [82–85]. A good contrasting agent for MRI is selected by looking at its longitudinal relaxivity (r1/mM-1s-1), [86]. A lysine-based group of dendritic contrast agents, named Gadomer-17 and Gd(III) DTPA-24-cascade-polymer, was developed [87–91]. To cater the needs of a target specific MRI, specialised contrasting agents were developed which binds only to a specific region or tissue, according to the disease [92]. For molecular MRI, to enhance the local concentration of the receptors, several targeting agents are used [93]. Oligonucleotides [93], proteins [94–96], carbohydrates [97–99], antibodies [100], oligopeptides [94, 101], and folic acid [102, 103] are added to the periphery. These target specific MRI contrasting agents were tested for its efficacy in *in vivo* conditions by injecting it to mice with ovarian tumors and expressing the folate receptors. When this dendritic contrasting agent was used, the signal improved significantly, while there was no signal when checked in folate receptor-negative tumours [103, 104].

Use of Dendrimers as Computed Tomography (CT) Agents

Very few studies have employed dendrimers as an imaging tool. One of the reasons is that we need a high dose of contrasting agents which ultimately leads to toxicity. But there are a few situations where iodinated dendrimers are used, for instance, in CT angiography where the blood flow in the blood vessels is visualized or neuro-angiography for suspected stroke, or pulmonary-angiography for suspected pulmonary embolus. In these cases contrasting agents with low molecular weight can slip through the intravascular compartment but the pulmonary agents with high molecular weight will stay back in the vessels [105].

Dendrimers Used as Transmission Electron Microscopy (TEM) Agents

The new class of dendrimer known as dendrimer-entrapped metal NPs is used for TEM since the high electron density properties of noble metals like silver and gold make TEM imaging easier. Gold/PAMAM dendrimer composites were tested in both *in vitro* and *in vivo* conditions [106]. In both conditions, it is efficient in making the visualization process successful. Silver/dendrimer nanocomposites were also developed as a potential molecule for TEM imaging [106].

Miscellaneous NPs for Imaging

Calcium Phosphate NPs

Calcium phosphate NPs are used in different fields of therapeutic biology due to their lower toxicity level. They have been used as a drug-delivering agent for antibiotics, anti-inflammatory drugs, bisphosphonates, and growth factors, and as a gene-delivering agent in association with DNA (cell transfection), RNA, siRNA, and miRNA [107, 108]. They are also used in hard tissue formation like bone and teeth [109]. They have received attention because of their biocompatibility, biodegradability, and non-viral properties, and also their incompatibility with microbial degradation [110]. Calcium phosphate is also used in biomedical imaging after doping lanthanides or surface-functionalization with organic dyes. Different lanthanide ions give different colours such as europium—red light—and terbium—green light [111]. A bioresorbable calcium NPs has been synthesized which gives fluorophore indocyanine green (ICG) on exposure to NIR, and is used to detect breast tumours [13, 112].

Lipid-Based NPs

Lipid-based NPs such as liposomes, nanostructured lipid carriers (NLC), and solid lipid NPs (SLN) are extensively used as analytic and therapeutic agents. These particles are preferably used as theranostic agents because they can transport both hydrophilic and hydrophobic agents. They have low or no toxicity and a prolonged half-life [13].

   i. Liposomes are bilayered vesicles, composed of lipids like phospholipids or cholesterols. They encapsulate the delivering agent forming a micelle-like structure which ensures the stability of the delivering agent, decreases the fluidity of NPs, and increases the permeability.

   ii. Solid lipid NPs remain at a solid state at both room and body temperature. The lipids used in the formation of SLN are highly purified fatty acids, triglycerides, and glycerides, generally having a low potential for toxicity. They show physical stability, site-specific recognition, low toxicity, cost-effectiveness, ease to manufacture, minimum degradation of encircled particles, and controlled release, but have moderate drug-storing capacity and drug explosion due to crystallization. These are used to transfer agents like quantum dots, technetium-99, super paramagnetic iron oxides, and ^{64}Cu. The NPs can pass through the blood–brain barrier, so they can be used as a CNS MRI diagnostic agent. SLNs with QDs are used in the visualization of cancer cells. ^{64}Cu radiolabelled SLNs can be useful in PET imaging. They are also used in the diagnosis of rheumatoid arthritis by binding the anti-CD64 antibody to cell surface receptors on rheumatoid arthritis-infected macrophages. So the SLNs act as a good theranostic agent due to their biodegradability and biocompatibility.

   iii. NLCs were introduced by Muller et al., and they are the modifications of SLN. These are composed of both solid and liquid lipids and can overcome the limitations of SLNs. The particle size is similar to SLNs, that is 10–1,000 nm. NLCs show site-specific targeting, surface modification, controlled drug release, low toxicity, more physical stability, and minimum degradation and can be loaded with hydrophobic and hydrophilic drugs. They are used as a drug carrier in leukaemia, tumour targeting, psoriasis, antifungal activity, and medical imaging.

Perfluorocarbon NPs (PFCN)

PFC NPs are non-toxic, non-volatile, non-degradable, and inert paramagnetic agents, allowing them to be used as contrast and drug delivery agents. Structurally they are derived from hydrocarbons but instead of hydrogen atoms, fluorine atoms are present [113]. They can carry a sufficient amount of oxygen, so act as blood substitutes. Liquid PFC is used for organ preservation. A PFC nanoparticle comprises a liquid perfluorocarbon core encapsulated with monolayer lipid with a diameter 150–250 nm. The surface charge of PFCN depends on the nature of phospholipids used. The surface lipid layer can be covalently bonded with peptides, antibodies, and peptidomimetics [114, 115].

The PFC NPs have much use in molecular imaging. As the body does not contain fluorine naturally, PFC can use as contrast agents in MRI [116, 117] to detect mammary tumours [118], cellular tracking [119, 120], atherosclerosis [121], and imaging of hypoxia [122]. Chelated lanthanides linked PFCN [123] and gadolinium added PFC are utilized as contrast agents in MRI. They are also used in ultrasound [124, 125], fluorescence, SPECT, and CT scanning [126]. They have a half-life from 3 to 42 hours, no kidney toxicity, and mild side effects like fever and flu-like symptoms, so they exhibit a good safety profile [13, 127].

Polyelectrolyte Complex NPs (PECNs)

Polymers that have a negative or positive charge at neutral pH are called polyelectrolyte [13]. A polyelectrolyte complex is formed due to electrostatic interaction between two oppositely charged polyions [128]. PECNs are used in biomedical imaging because they show low toxicity, high compatibility, and more biodegradability [129]. The PECNs are manufactured in two ways: bottom-up and bottom-down techniques. The bottom-up method is widely used and the polymeric cations and anions form electrostatic bonds in an aqueous medium [130–132]. It depends on some intrinsic (chemical nature, charge, and weight) and extrinsic factors [133]. The extrinsic factors also depend on pH, temperature, ionic strength, etc., and mixing processes. The bottom-down method includes sonication, homogenization, and ultra-high pressure. NPs developed by this method are suitable for easy transfer but the chemical degradation of materials may be seen due to the application of high energy [134]. PEC capsules can be produced by the aggregation of oppositely charged ions in the colloidal substrate using a layer-by-layer technique [135]. PECNs are used in drug delivery and imaging techniques. The PEC prepared from chitosan shows potential use in drug delivery [136]. These PECs are used to deliver small particles, large proteins, peptides, and RNAs [137, 138]. They are also used in biomedical imaging such as benzothiadiazole-conjugated PEC [139], hyperbranched conjugated PEC [140], chitosan-coated manganese zinc ferrite [141], gadolinium incorporated PEC, and fluorescence probe (AlexaFluor 750) incorporated low-molecular-mass poly hydrochloride PEC [142].

NPS That Improve Imaging in Certain Instruments

Magnetic Resonance Imaging (MRI)

MRI is an imaging technique used for the recognition of disease. It is a nuclear magnetic resonance (NMR) that uses nuclei of unpaired electrons to produce a magnetic resonance image [143, 144]. The nuclei used are generally hydrogen nuclei because of their abundance in water and fat. These unpaired electrons act like a tiny magnet that rotates around its axis in the influence of the earth's magnetic field. In the MRI scanner, the protons' axes are all lined up; when additional radio waves are added to the magnetic field the protons rotate from their position which can be 90° or 180°. When the radio frequency switches off the nuclei return back to their resting state which emits a signal and is detected by sensors and used to create MR images (Figure 5.1). This results in the formation of two independent relaxation parameters, the transverse (T1) and longitudinal (T2) relaxation time. Many contrasting agents used in MRI for contrast enhancement are classified under three categories. The first one is T1-weighted

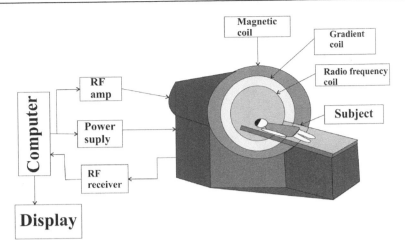

Figure 5.1 A graphical set up for a patient undergoing an MRI check-up.

contrast agents which are generally paramagnetic materials that shorten the T1 relaxation time and improve bright contrast on T1-weighted image. The MRI contrast agents used in medicines are under this category such as gadolinium (Gd^{3+}) [145]. This represents positive contrasts. The second type is T2-weighted contrasting agents, and they are super paramagnetic and shorten the T2 relaxation time and form dark contrast on T2-weighted images. T2 contrast agents are super magnetic iron oxides, which main component is magnetite (Fe_3O_4) or maghemite (Fe_2O_3). This represents negative contrasts. The third type is dual-weighted contrast agents, which enable both T1- and T2-weighted contrast agents, e.g., gadolinium oxides (Gd_2O_3) [146]. Because of the presence of high amounts of water, fats, and carbohydrate, the hydrogen MRI are noisy (have more signals in the background). So to overcome this limit, heteronuclear MRI atoms such as ^{13}C, ^{23}Na, ^{17}O, ^{31}P, ^{15}N, and ^{19}F have been developed [147, 148]. Among these, ^{19}F is used in cell tracking, lung imaging, and tumour labelling [149, 150].

Criteria Used to Design NPs as MRI Contrast Agents

i. The first is a magnetic particle with surface modification as a prerequisite due to its simple structure, e.g., super magnetic iron oxide NPs (SPIO) [151].

ii. In the next one, in the core there is magnetic material and organic or inorganic materials on the shell. Examples include micelles and dendrimers [152, 153]. In this type of nanoparticle, the size, solubility, and biosafety need to be taken into consideration.

iii. The third structure is a vector with magnetic materials on the surface or a ligand to connect with other NPs. Such surface modification contrast to MRI and the main nanoparticle helps in fluorescence imaging, CT imaging, and drug loading [146].

iv. The fourth one is the mixed structure with magnetic material coated on either surface. An example is liposomal-gadolinium [154].

Computed Tomography (CT)

CT is a radiography imaging method that uses high-energy electromagnetic radiation to produce transverse and three-dimensional pictures of internal structures without sectioning. It was introduced in the 1970s [155]. Although it shows high radiation, it is still widely used

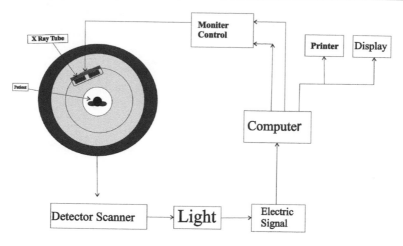

Figure 5.2 A complete set up to image under computed tomography.

in diagnosis because it has higher resolution and efficiency, faster examination, and low cost [156]. The body is passed through the loop like a CT scanner to obtain the images, and it spins around the body. The machine has an X-ray source and opposite to it, an X-ray detector is present which detects X-rays from the body. Scintillator photo diode detectors are used (Figure 5.2). The scintillator collects X-rays that are converted to light, which are then converted into an electric signal by photo diode [156]. This electric signal is then organized by a processer to form transverse images or sections called tomograms.

Contrast agents perform a major role in CT imaging. The most used contrasting agent is iodine but it shows renal toxicity, anaphylaxis, and fast clearance. So NPs are used to enhance the efficiency of CT scans. Two types of CT contrast agents are formed depending on the structure of NPs.

i. The principal one is iodine-based in which the iodine is present in the core of the nanoparticle like liposomal iodine. This lowers the risk associated with iodine. These are used to detect tumour vessels [157].

ii. The second is metal-based which is metal with a high X-ray attenuation coefficient. Examples of metals include gold, titanium oxide, and zirconium oxide. Gold NPs are used for the imaging of blood flow and prostate cancer [22]. Zirconium dioxide is used to image tumours. Gold NPs are commonly used because they show more efficiency than liposomal iodine. AuNPs can detect malignant glioma by trailing on Mesenchymal stem cells [146].

Ultrasound (US)

Ultrasound or sonography is a non-invasive, real-time imaging technique that uses sound waves [158]. Instead of X-rays, it uses high-frequency sound waves, which enter the body from a transducer through the gel (on the body). The reflected sound waves captured by the probe and image can be generated by a computer analyzing the waves [159]. The shorter wavelengths generate accurate images (Figure 5.3) [146]. US is used to diagnose heart conditions, causes of infection, swelling in internal organs, checking the baby of pregnant women, guiding during biopsies, etc. [159], and the movement of internal organs and blood vessels. Transrectal US

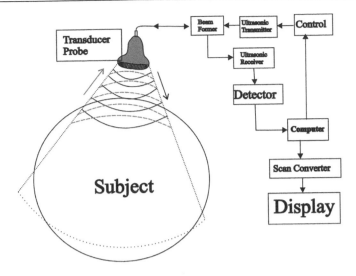

Figure 5.3 A comprehensive set up for image analysis under ultrasound.

(TRUS) is used to diagnose and perform biopsies of prostate cancer [160], and endoscopic US diagnoses gastrointestinal tumours like pancreatic tumours [161]. The contrast agents used in US range from 1 to 8 μm in size and have low stability; to overcome this demerit nowadays nanoparticles are used.

With the small size of the NPs and their surface-modifying characteristic, they can achieve better targeting to lesions. The NPs used in US imaging are divided into three types based on their composition.

  i. The first and most common type is microbubble. These use gases like carbon dioxide, sulphur hexafluoride, nitrogen, and perfluorocarbon, for strong reflection. The NPs used are silica NPs, liposomes, and polymer NPs.
 ii. The second one is solid-based nanoparticles, smaller than microbubbles but with high scattering signals. Due to their small size, they can be easily accumulated in target sites. An example is rattle-typed mesoporous silica nanostructures used in tumour diagnosis.
iii. The third type is liquid-based nanoparticles, which use lower speed sound emission to generate the signal. An example is perfluoroocytyl bromide nanoparticles.

The gases are loaded in the core of NPs by three different means:

  i. In the first method, the gases (nitrogen, perfluorocarbon, CO_2, and sulphur hexafluoride) are loaded in the core of NPs.
 ii. The second method is the phase transition method. In this method the watery substance existing in the core of NPs is stimulated to form gas by sound waves, when it reaches the target lesions. It is done using AuNP-coated/perfluorocarbon-encapsulated mesoporous silica nanocapsules.
iii. In the third method, carbonate is used to create a chemical reaction in which gas is generated. Carbonate is insoluble at neutral pH, so easily accumulated in the tumours. Then carbon dioxide is generated from carbonate in the acidic environment of tumours, which then generates a signal. Examples are ammonium bicarbonate and poly NPs.

Examples of NPs used in US are PLA-Herceptin, C3F8-filled PLGA exosome-like silica NP, PFC-NP (C4F10), silica-coated NPs, FA-PEG-CS, and perfluorooctyl bromide nanocore [146].

Positron Emission Tomography (PET)

PET is a part of nuclear medicine [162], that involves the use of radioactive elements to study tissue and organ functions. The PET produces real time images with high sensitivity and high tissue penetration. Radioisotopes used in PET are 11C,^{15}N, ^{15}O, and ^{18}F. The imaging technique involves the administration of tracer elements in the bloodstream, intravenously. After the accumulation of radioactive elements in the tissue and organs, an annihilation reaction occurs as a result of which the tracers emit positrons that collide with electrons in the tissue and produce energy (Figure 5.4). Then these radioactive emissions (photons) are detected by the PET camera which is then converted into an electric signal within 10–40 minutes. For example: to detect the glucose consumption by different body parts, radiolabelled 18-fluorodeoxyglucose was used to check the glucose uptake [163]. The PET scan detects tumours, cancer, strokes, dementia (by studying blood flow and oxygen consumption), and Parkinson's disease (by tracking dopamine).

The nucleotides with a higher half-life and in the form of NPs are used for PET analysis. The NPs include copper-64, indium-111, iodine-123, 125, and 131, and gold-198 and 199. NPs are synthesized by a translational method, using poly (4-vinylphenol) (PVPh) polymer radiolabelled I-124, and surface-fabricated antibodies pointing endothelium are used for stability. Tri-modality NPs like starch-based iron oxide and dextran-decorated iron oxide NPs were used in MRI, PET, and fluorescence imaging. Zr-89 radiolabelled dextran NPs are utilized in macrophage imaging. Radioactive liposomes labelled with Lu-177 were used to wipe out tumour cells [146].

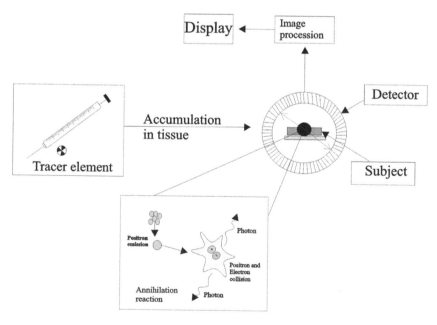

Figure 5.4 An image depicting analysis of defects under PET scan.

Single-Photon Emission Computed Tomography (SPECT)

It is based on nuclear medicine technology and the advancement of tomographic imaging. The technique of SPECT is similar to PET but it uses gamma rays. The imaging procedure is the same as the nuclear medicine imaging technique. The radiopharmaceutical element is administered into the patient's body, which gets accumulated in tissue and organs. These radionucleotides then emit gamma rays which pass through a scintillation camera. The camera is made up of a lead collimator that localizes the gamma-ray photons and converts them into lower-energy photons. These are then converted into electric signals by a photomultiplier tube. The SPECT takes 2D images from different angles which combine to form a 3D image (Figure 5.5) [164]. The radionucleotides in SPECT have a higher half-life than in PET. The commonly used nucleotide is technetium-99 with a half-life of 6 hours.

SPECT scanning is used to generate cardiac and brain imaging (as it can detect blood flow), tumour imaging, thyroid imaging, leukocyte infection imaging, scintigraphy of bones, neuroimaging, etc. ^{111}In-labelled annexin A5-CCPM is used to detect tumour apoptosis. ^{99m}Tc-labelled superparamagnetic iron oxide [165] and radiolabelled iron oxide NPs are applied as dual modalities in SPECT/MRI scanners [166]. SPECT in combination with CT gives anatomical and functional information [167]. Chlorotoxin peptide-functionalized polyethyleneimine-entrapped gold NPs are used in the detection and therapy of malignant glioma (a lethal type of brain cancer) in SPECT/CT imaging [168]. Lipid-calcium phosphate NPs are used in SPECT/CT imaging of lymph node metastases [169]. Iodine-125-labelled silver NPs are also used in SPECT imaging [146, 170].

Optical Imaging (OI)

Optical imaging involves series of techniques that are based on the emission of electromagnetic light such as UV, visible spectrum, and IR. OI mostly takes account of bioluminescence and fluorescence. In fluorescence imaging, the fluorophores are excited

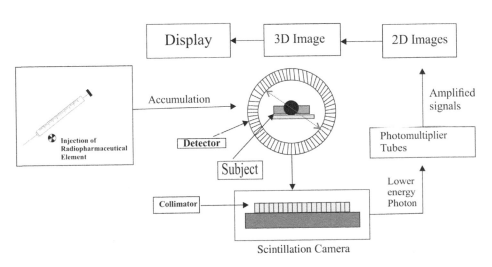

Figure 5.5 A set up for image analysis under SPECT scan.

by external light with appropriate wave length. On excitation, the fluorophore molecules jump from the ground state to the excited state by absorbing energy. Then some part of the absorbed energy is released on its way back to the ground state, and this shows fluorescence (Figure 5.6). The emitted fluorescence has a longer wavelength than the incident light. The probes used as fluorophore are generally organic dyes, quantum dots [171], green fluorescent protein [172], phalloidin, luciferase, DAPI [173], cyanine dyes [174, 175], etc. Near-infrared fluorescence (NIRF) is used to image deeper tissues [146, 176]. Bioluminescence is the light generated by the reaction between the substrate of interest and luciferase enzyme. This enzyme oxidizes its substrate in the presence of oxygen and ATP and emits light with a broad spectrum. After intraperitoneal injection, the luciferase can cross the blood–tissue barrier and reach the brain and placenta. Its half-life is 60 min which gives sufficient time for imaging. *Pyrophorus plagiophthalamus* (click beetle) luciferase shows green-orange; *Renilla* (sea pansy) and *Gaussia* (marine copepod) luciferases produce blue light after oxidation [177].

In multimodality imaging, OI plays a major role as it is a small, easy to conjugate, and robust system. MR/OI contrast agents are gadolinium-based probes that help in cell tracking [178], and iron oxide probes [179]. PET/OI probes are produced by the direct conjugation of radiotracer and fluorophores or through carrier systems. A SPECT/OI probe is also produced by chelation, and an example is a single amino acid chelate. US/OI probes are like microbubbles which are made by adding OI fluorescent dye to pre-formed bubbles or during the synthesis of bubbles. This is used to study biodistribution and clearance of bubbles. Multimodal CT/OI contrast agents are utilized to study anatomical, functional, and molecular information at high resolution. Glycol chitosan-coated gold NPs conjugated with matrix metalloproteinase (MMP)-cleavable peptides are used as CT/OI probes [177].

Many NP OI probes are used in biomedical imaging. For tumour imaging, oleic acid chitosan-coated iron oxides [180], HiLyte Fluor-647 loaded hyaluronic acid gold NPs [181],

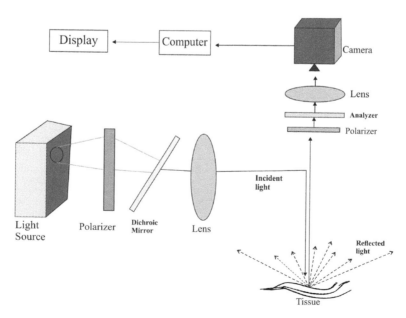

Figure 5.6 Analysis of defective regions under optical imaging.

and Cy5.5 labelled SPIONs [182] (brain tumours) are utilized. HEPA-Au NPs are applied as CT/OI contrast agents in liver imaging. NIR-dye labelled probes can detect several receptors in human breast cancer xenograft [183]. QD agitated probes are used in DNA hybridization studies (CdSe/ZnS QD) [184, 185], the recognition of genomic alterations of cancer, the detection of infectious bacterial strains (phage conjugated streptavidin-coated QDs) [186], the detection of toxins (antibody-conjugated CdSe/ZnS) [187], etc. OI has several advantages such as it is user-friendly and low cost, bioluminescence and fluorescence both can be done, it does not require extra processing, and high-speed data collection [188]. With the use of nanoparticles, OI will improve further as an imaging tool.

Photoacoustic Imaging (PAI)

PAI is the hybrid of optical imaging in addition to spatial resolution ultrasound. It is also known as thermoacoustic or optoacoustic imaging. It uses the emission of acoustic energy at megahertz frequency which is the result of the absorption of electromagnetic energy by endogenous or exogenous chromophores. These photoacoustic waves are detected by an ultrasound transducer that maps the electromagnetic radiation energy absorption properties. From this, the PA signal structure and properties of tissue can be concluded, known as PA depth profiling (Figure 5.7). For imaging more complicated structures PA tomography is used, which is also known as optoacoustic or thermoacoustic tomography (OAT/TAT). The energy used is non-ionizing waves which do not create any health hazards. These can form images of high ultrasound resolution. Recently PAI has been used for photoacoustic tomography and photoacoustic microscopy (PAM). The PAM includes an ultrasonic detector with a confocal optical illumination. This improves the signal-to-noise ratio [189].

PAI is primarily used for tumour detection, the identification of metastatic lymph nodes, therapeutic monitoring, and molecular characterization. Both endogenous (haemoglobin) and exogenous (organic dyes) contrast agents are utilized in PAI [190]. Endogenous contrast agents can help to study tumour angiogenesis, lipid distribution, characterization of melanoma cells, etc. Among exogenous contrast agents, NIR dyes are mostly used. An example is indocyanine green (ICG) which is used in cancer research.

NPs can act as contrast agents due to their ability to image deeper tissue with enhanced contrast, large target binding site, flexibility, easy targeting peptides, and antibodies.

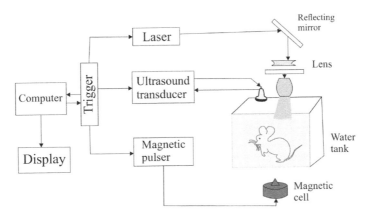

Figure 5.7 A thorough set up for the analysis of defects under photoacoustic imaging.

According to their light absorption nature, they are divided into two types: (a) particles based on surface plasmon resonance (SPR) and (b) dye-containing NPs [191]. SPR involves gold NPs which show high biocompatibility, stability, and active targeting. On absorption of energy, GNPs oscillate around the core called plasmon, which is then converted to heat and detected by PAI. It is used to target angiogenic tumour vasculature. RGD-modified GNPs slow tumour accumulation [192]. Antibody-conjugated GNPs can target extracellular receptors. Dye-containing NPs use NIR organic dyes to enhance absorption. ICG was conjugated with NPs and used as a contrast agent due to its non-toxic property [191]. The targeting of integrin for angiogenesis study is done by using RGD peptides attached to SWNTs [193]. Porphyrin-palladium hydride MOF NPs are utilized in cancer therapy [194]. RGD-conjugated silica-coated gold nanorods help in gastric cancer imaging [195].

Multiphoton Imaging

In the multiphoton imaging technique, multiple low-energy photons interact with a fluorophore at the same time or the time interval is less than 10^{-8} sec, exciting it to the higher transition state. A high number of photon incidents are required to generate nonlinear interaction. Each exciting photon contributes to the excitation of a molecule. Upon its way back it emits a fluorescence signal, which has a shorter wavelength than the excitation light (Figure 5.8). This signal is detected by a confocal microscope [196]. The detectors used can collect scattering signals and can give two to three times deeper images in comparison with confocal microscopy. The multiphoton imaging also shows

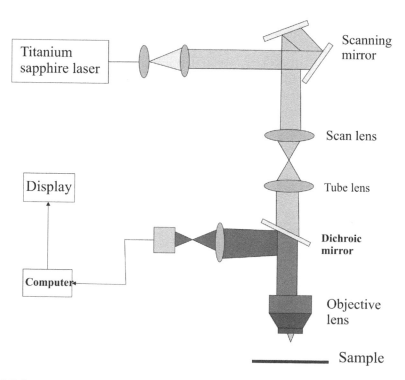

Figure 5.8 A systematic set up for image analysis using multiphoton imaging.

flexibility, for example two-photon absorption wave length for rhodamine is 700 nm which is same for DAPI, so both can be imaged [197]. This multiphoton imaging method helps to study Alzheimer's disease [198], tumours [199], cholesterol uptake [200], secretion, NADH metabolism, lipid phase, membranes, plant structures, calcium and sodium dynamics [201], and neural plasticity [202]. NPs used in multiphoton imaging are folate-modified silicon carbide NPs in cancer cell detection [203], cadmium sulphide NPs [204], gold NPs in tumours [205], antibody-conjugated GNPs in breast cancer [206], and conjugated polymer NPs in endothelial cell imaging [207].

Radiography

This is an imaging technique that involves X-rays. The X-rays are high-frequency waves that are reflected, absorbed, or traversed through the body on the incident. The X-ray is generated in an X-ray tube containing a cathode (tungsten filament) and an anode. In this process, the patient is positioned at the target place and the X-rays pass through the body. Collimators are used to define the X-ray field. The X-rays through the body strike at the receptor present behind the body. In conventional radiography, the receptor is composed of two layers of polyester bed sheet in between silver bromide crystal emulsion (Figure 5.9). The latent image generated after X-ray detection requires further processing by developers (chemicals) and undergoes fixing, washing, and drying to create an image. In computed radiography, X-rays hit a photosensitive phosphor plate, and electrons of phosphor particles form a latent image. This latent image is processed by laser to form a visible image. Digital radiography has different chemicals which form electric signals, and the image is generated by a computer in real-time [208]. The image depends on the position, size, and structure of the target, and X-ray exposure time. This technique is used to screen tumours [209], breast cancer [210], and pneumonia [211], and during joint injection [212], the insertion of stents [213], etc. Gold NPs [214, 215] and gadolinium [216] NPs are generally used in radiography imaging.

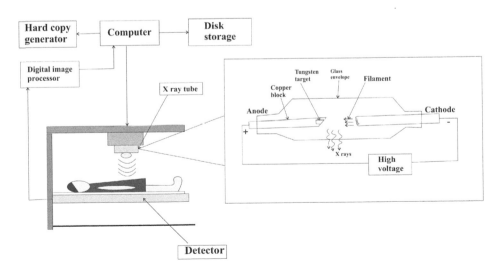

Figure 5.9 Analysis of an image using a radiography technique.

Scintigraphy

This is a two-dimensional imaging technique in which radiopharmaceutical contrast agents are used to generate images. The procedure is similar to SPECT. In this, the contrast agent is introduced into the patients, and the images are taken four to five days after the injection. This lowers background activity and generates high-quality images. Gamma scintillation cameras are used to take images [217]. Scintigraphy imaging is used in adrenal imaging [217, 218], renal cortical scintigraphy in the diagnosis of acute pyelonephritis [219], in coronary artery disease [220], Parkinson's disease [221], skeletal scintigraphy for the detection of injuries [222], and many more applications in biomedical identification and prognosis. NPs used in scintigraphy are small unimolar liposomes and reverse-phase vesicles [223], bromocriptine conjugated chitosan NPs [47], lipid-based NPs (in brain pharmacokinetics) [224], AuNPs (in renal clearance) [225], curcumin-containing chitosan NPs (for colon drug delivery and ulcerative colitis treatment) [226], curcumin loaded SLNs (in liver-spleen imaging) [227], folate conjugated iron oxides (for tumours) [228], levofloxine [229] and dorzolamide [230] (for glaucoma) loaded chitosan NPs, ropinirole loaded mucoadhesive NPs (for the brain) [231], piperine loaded chitosan NPs (for brain targeting in Alzheimer's) [232], etc.

NPs Used as an Imaging Probe for Diagnosis

Many NPs are used as probes for several diagnoses such as (a) cell labelling and tracking, (b) for contrast enhancement in the blood, (c) for analysis of blood vascular systems (MPS), and (d) for imaging hyperthermia treatment.

NP as a Probe for Cell Labelling and Tracking

Cells can be labelled directly as well as indirectly. In the case of indirect labelling reporter genes with imaging markers are introduced *in-vivo* transplantation [233–235]. For direct cell labelling NPs are incubated with the cells having phagocytic activity [233, 236–238]. In direct cell labelling the NPs get diluted when the cell population is higher [238, 239]. Direct labelling does not allow us to count cell viability, proliferation, or cell death. For MRI gadolinium (paramagnetic) or iron oxide (paramagnetic) NPs are used for direct labelling. Gold NPs are used for labelling in CT [240], manganese particles for MR imaging [241, 242], and positron-labelled NPs are used for PET [242]. The amount of NPs internalized by the cell along with the pulse sequence determines the sensitivity of MR imaging-based cell tracking. Patients with traumatic brain injury were administered NPs to label autologous neural stem cells, and later the cell movements were recorded [243]. Still, further study is needed to use the NPs for clinical trials.

As a Blood Pool Contrasting Agent

The blood pool contrasting agents help to visualize smaller or larger blood vessels which are used in diagnostic purposes for many diseases such as cancer, thrombosis, atherosclerosis, venous insufficiency, and vascular inflammation. Mainly soft and hard (metal-based) nanomaterials are used for this purpose. The soft nano-sized blood pool contrasting agents have a size of 0–150 nm, and for CT imaging, iodinated liposomes [244-246], micelles [247, 248], or polymers [249, 250] are used. Metal-based NPs also give excellent contrast in CT imaging. One of the examples is barium ytterbium-fluor NPs with silica and polyethylene glycol coating [251]. Gold NPs are an efficient candidate for the blood pool contrasting agent because they have excellent targeting of the diseased and the defective tissue. Research groups have used gold NPs with gum Arabic as the capping agent. Initial CT attenuations using phantoms were 80 and 140 kVp. These NPs were injected in a swine model, and their biodistribution was detected in the lungs, spleen, and liver [20].

Imaging in MPS

The reticuloendothelial system also known as mononuclear phagocyte system (MPS) consists of the spleen, lymphatics, and the liver. The MPS can be easily visualized by the NPs due to the high number of macrophages existing in them (Kupffer cells in the liver) [252]. MPS can be imaged using MRI [253–257], optical aging [258], CT [245, 246, 248], photoacoustic imaging [259], and single-photon emission CT (SPECT) [260]. A group of researchers have tried a technique for sentinel lymph node detection where probes were inserted into the vicinity of the tumour and then the NPs get accumulated in the lymph nodes. NPs like iron oxide NP, QDs, gold nanocages, and microtubules are injected for the detection of lymph nodes in tumours [261]. Iron oxide NPs (USPIO) are more suitable for MR imaging due to their paramagnetic nature. More importantly, SPIO and the USPIO nanoparticles are cleaned up via macrophages and in the liver Kupffer cells if the liver is in a functional state. But in a diseased liver the macrophages gets damaged which reduces the uptake of SPIO and this results in a bright spot in the image denoting the diseased area. Moreover the Kupffer cells are exiled by the tumour cells in the MR images and clearly the tumour region can be distinguished from the unaffected liver with diminished signalling [253, 262]. The metastasis of colorectal cancer has been visualised using SPIO-enhanced liver imaging by MR, and it was found to be highly sensitive [263, 264]. One disadvantage of this process can be false readings in the case of hepatocellular carcinoma where Kupffer cells statically exist in the early stages and can uptake the NPs. This case is also seen in hepatic adenomas [265]. MR imaging with iron oxide NPs is also used in model organisms and patients to visualize insulitis which is a symptom of the early progression of type I diabetes in which the autoimmune reaction of the body will destroy the islet cells. In the inflammatory reaction that follows this autoimmune reaction, vessel leakiness takes place [266]. The nanoparticles can be injected to the patient and through the blood circulation it can reach the leaky blood vessel and then leak out from it and end up floating in the surrounding tissue. This is then taken up by the existing macrophages [267].

Imaging-Guided Hyperthermia Treatment

NPs can be used to treat hyperthermia patients since they can absorb energy and convert them into heat. This is done by radiation with acoustic [268, 269] as well as electromagnetic [270] waves and with light [271–273]. The major disadvantage of this technique is that we cannot ensure the localisation of sufficient amount of NPs in the tissue of target. To overcome this problem with catheter-based local arterial injections, systemic intra-venous injections are used [274]. This imaging-based hyperthermia treatment is beneficial for malignant brain tumour patients as the therapeutic options for this are limited (apart from the conventional methods like surgery, chemotherapy, and radiotherapy). Magnetic NPs were injected under CT control and localized into the glioblastomas and then heated by applying the magnetic forces [270]. This method is effective and increases the overall survival rate of glioblastoma patients, hence, opening a new opportunity for the theranostic approach to treatment [270].

Advantages and Disadvantages of NPs Used for Imaging

NPs used in molecular imaging have led to the discovery of novel agents used for therapeutics and bioimaging. The pros and cons of NPs are determined by toxicity, pharmacokinetics, biocompatibility, and immunogenicity. The advantages of using NPs in imaging are (a) the increased surface area to volume ratio with a decreased diameter, which helps to form functionally active particles targeting cells or tissues [275]; and (b) the small size of NPs which allows surface modification and allows them to easily pass through different biological barriers. For example, gadolinium-conjugated polyamidoamine is used in mice model [276] and carbohydrate-functionalized iron oxide is used in the CD62 imaging of rat brain by MRI [277]. The multimodal NPs have opened the doors for multiple imaging. These NPs are used for the detection of inflammation, tumours, apoptosis, and atherosclerosis. The fabricated iron oxide with infrared fluorophore Cy5.5 and a 35-amino acid peptide from the scorpion *Leiurus quinquestriatus* is used in brain cancer visualization [278]. NPs can also quantify enzyme activity, gene expression, protein-protein interaction, receptor density, and the activity of ion channels. Gene expression can be visualized by using specific promoters, e.g., 9-(4-18F-fluoro-3-[hydroxymethyl]butyl-)guanine and 18F-fluoropenciclovir in herpes virus for thymidine kinase transgene expression [279]. By using fluorescent probes enzyme activity can be observed, e.g., to quantify cathepsin B activity, Cy3.5 and Cy5.5 attached cathepsin B-sensitive and -resistant peptides were applied [280].

The NPs used for bioimaging also have some disadvantages. The NPs may act as phagocytic cells and can be destroyed by macrophages or, accumulated in the liver, also can alter surface properties of plasma protein by interacting with them [275]. Serum-coated NPs can pass through biological barriers and can be accumulated in reticuloendothelial cells. For example, chlorotoxin modified iron oxides pass through the blood–brain barrier and can image tumours [281]. The accumulation and nonspecific phagocytosis of NPs by the reticuloendothelial system, and macrophage-related disease imaging, results in loss of specificity and toxicity building. To overcome this, many modifications were made using PEG [281] and polysaccharides dextran [282] and several approaches were made, but none was completely effective. NPs can induce toxicity from themselves or the individual components they are made of. For example, QDs release cadmium which is toxic to humans, and gadolinium chelates are nephrotoxic [283, 284]. These NPs show cytotoxicity [285, 286], immune response [287], accumulation in lungs [288], passing through the blood–brain barrier and invoke degeneration and necrosis in neurons [289] and oxidative stress generation [285]. Dendrimers are low-priced and simple but also show toxic effects [290]. Many particles also accumulate in tumour tissue and create an enhanced permeability and retention (EPR) effect [291]. Although NPs have both effects, the negative effect can be modified to reduce the toxicity and to be widely used for biomedical imaging.

References

1. Satpathy, A., Ranjan R., Priyadarsini S., Gupta S., Mathur P., Mishra M. (2019) Diagnostic Imaging Techniques in Oral Diseases. In: Shukla A. (eds) *Medical Imaging Methods*. Springer, Singapore. https://doi.org/10.1007/978-981-13-9121-7_3.

2. Tempany, C.M. and B.J. McNeil, Advances in biomedical imaging. *JAMA*, 2001. **285**(5): p. 562–567.

3. Yigit, M.V., A. Moore, and Z. Medarova, Magnetic nanoparticles for cancer diagnosis and therapy. *Pharmaceutical Research*, 2012. **29**(5): p. 1180–1188.

4. Jakhmola, A., N. Anton, and T.F. Vandamme, Inorganic nanoparticles based contrast agents for X-ray computed tomography. *Advanced Healthcare Materials*, 2012. **1**(4): p. 413–431.

5. Wahajuddin, S.A., Superparamagnetic iron oxide nanoparticles: Magnetic nanoplatforms as drug carriers. *International Journal of Nanomedicine*, 2012. **7**: p. 3445.

6. Kiessling, F., B. Morgenstern, and C. Zhang, Contrast agents and applications to assess tumor angiogenesis in vivo by magnetic resonance imaging. *Current Medicinal Chemistry*, 2007. **14**(1): p. 77–91.

7. Priyadarsini, S., et al., Oral administration of graphene oxide nano-sheets induces oxidative stress, genotoxicity, and behavioral teratogenicity in Drosophila melanogaster. *Environmental Science and Pollution Research*, 2019. **26**(19): p. 19560–19574.

8. Barik, B.K. and M. Mishra, Nanoparticles as a potential teratogen: A lesson learnt from fruit fly. *Nanotoxicology*, 2019. **13**(2): p. 258–284.

9. Mallick, T., et al., Carbazole analog anchored fluorescent silica nanoparticle showing enhanced biocompatibility and selective sensing ability towards biomacromolecule. *Dyes and Pigments*, 2020. **173**: p. 107994.

10. Mishra, M. and M. Panda, Reactive oxygen species: The root cause of nanoparticle-induced toxicity in Drosophila melanogaster. *Free Radical Research*, 2021: **55**(6): p. 671–687.

11. Al-Jamal, W.T., et al., Functionalized-quantum-dot–liposome hybrids as multimodal nanoparticles for cancer. *Small*, 2008. **4**(9): p. 1406–1415.

12. Cai, W. and X. Chen, Nanoplatforms for targeted molecular imaging in living subjects. *Small*, 2007. **3**(11): p. 1840–1854.

13. Nune, S.K., et al., Nanoparticles for biomedical imaging. *Expert Opinion on Drug Delivery*, 2009. **6**(11): p. 1175–1194.

14. Turkevich, J., P.C. Stevenson, and J. Hillier, A study of the nucleation and growth processes in the synthesis of colloidal gold. *Discussions of the Faraday Society*, 1951. **11**: p. 55–75.

15. Brust, M., et al., Synthesis of thiol-derivatised gold nanoparticles in a two-phase liquid–liquid system. *Journal of the Chemical Society, Chemical Communications*, 1994. **7**: p. 801–802.

16. Brust, M., et al., Synthesis and reactions of functionalised gold nanoparticles. *Journal of the Chemical Society, Chemical Communications*, 1995. **16**: p. 1655–1656.

17. Yu, S.-B. and A.D. Watson, Metal-based X-ray contrast media. *Chemical Reviews*, 1999. **99**(9): p. 2353–2378.

18. Blaszkiewicz, P., Synthesis of water-soluble ionic and nonionic iodinated X-ray contrast media. *Investigative Radiology*, 1994. **29**(Supplement 1): p. S51–S53.

19. Galperin, A., et al., Radiopaque iodinated polymeric nanoparticles for X-ray imaging applications. *Biomaterials*, 2007. **28**(30): p. 4461–4468.

20. Kattumuri, V., et al., Gum arabic as a phytochemical construct for the stabilization of gold nanoparticles: In vivo pharmacokinetics and X-ray-contrast-imaging studies. *Small*, 2007. **3**(2): p. 333–341.

21. Kim, D., et al., Antibiofouling polymer-coated gold nanoparticles as a contrast agent for in vivo X-ray computed tomography imaging. *Journal of the American Chemical Society*, 2007. **129**(24): p. 7661–7665.

22. Popovtzer, R., et al., Targeted gold nanoparticles enable molecular CT imaging of cancer. *Nano Letters*, 2008. **8**(12): p. 4593–4596.

23. Nikoobakht, B. and M.A. El-Sayed, Preparation and growth mechanism of gold nanorods (NRs) using seed-mediated growth method. *Chemistry of Materials*, 2003. **15**(10): p. 1957–1962.

24. Kim, D.E., et al., Hyperacute direct thrombus imaging using computed tomography and gold nanoparticles. *Annals of Neurology*, 2013. **73**(5): p. 617–625.

25. Ghann, W.E., et al., Syntheses and characterization of lisinopril-coated gold nanoparticles as highly stable targeted CT contrast agents in cardiovascular diseases. *Langmuir*, 2012. **28**(28): p. 10398–10408.

26. Zhang, Z., R.D. Ross, and R.K. Roeder, Preparation of functionalized gold nanoparticles as a targeted X-ray contrast agent for damaged bone tissue. *Nanoscale*, 2010. **2**(4): p. 582–586.

27. Wang, Y., et al., Label-free Au cluster used for in vivo 2D and 3D computed tomography of murine kidneys. *Analytical Chemistry*, 2015. **87**(1): p. 343–345.

28. Zhao, W., M.A. Brook, and Y. Li, Design of gold nanoparticle-based colorimetric biosensing assays. *ChemBioChem*, 2008. **9**(15): p. 2363–2371.

29. Elghanian, R., et al., Selective colorimetric detection of polynucleotides based on the distance-dependent optical properties of gold nanoparticles. *Science*, 1997. **277**(5329): p. 1078–1081.

30. Mirkin, C.A., Programming the assembly of two-and three-dimensional architectures with DNA and nanoscale inorganic building blocks. *Inorganic Chemistry*, 2000. **39**(11): p. 2258–2272.

31. Liu, J. and Y. Lu, Accelerated color change of gold nanoparticles assembled by DNAzymes for simple and fast colorimetric Pb2+ detection. *Journal of the American Chemical Society*, 2004. **126**(39): p. 12298–12305.

32. Li, H., et al., Colorimetric detection of immunoglobulin G by use of functionalized gold nanoparticles on polyethylenimine film. *Analytical and Bioanalytical Chemistry*, 2006. **384**(7–8): p. 1518–1524.

33. Lee, J.S., M.S. Han, and C.A. Mirkin, Colorimetric detection of mercuric ion (Hg2+) in aqueous media using DNA-functionalized gold nanoparticles. *Angewandte Chemie International Edition*, 2007. **46**(22): p. 4093–4096.

34. Stoff-Khalili, M., P. Dall, and D. Curiel, Gene therapy for carcinoma of the breast. *Cancer Gene Therapy*, 2006. **13**(7): p. 633–647.

35. Swiderek, P., Fundamental processes in radiation damage of DNA. *Angewandte Chemie International Edition*, 2006. **45**(25): p. 4056–4059.

36. Ray, P.C., et al., Gold nanoparticle based FRET for DNA detection. *Plasmonics*, 2007. **2**(4): p. 173–183.

37. Wierzbinski, K.R., et al., Potential use of superparamagnetic iron oxide nanoparticles for in vitro and in vivo bioimaging of human myoblasts. *Scientific Reports*, 2018. **8**(1): p. 1–17.

38. D'Amato, R., et al. Advances in the preparation of novel functionalized nanoparticles for bioimaging, in *2009 9th IEEE Conference on Nanotechnology (IEEE-NANO)*. 2009: IEEE.

39. Wagner, A.M., et al., Quantum dots in biomedical applications. *Acta Biomaterialia*, 2019. **94**: p. 44–63.

40. Mattoussi, H., G. Palui, and H.B. Na, Luminescent quantum dots as platforms for probing in vitro and in vivo biological processes. *Advanced Drug Delivery Reviews*, 2012. **64**(2): p. 138–166.

41. Smith, A.M., et al., Bioconjugated quantum dots for in vivo molecular and cellular imaging. *Advanced Drug Delivery Reviews*, 2008. **60**(11): p. 1226–1240.

42. Resch-Genger, U., et al., Quantum dots versus organic dyes as fluorescent labels. *Nature Methods*, 2008. **5**(9): p. 763.

43. Li, C., et al., In vivo real-time visualization of tissue blood flow and angiogenesis using Ag2S quantum dots in the NIR-II window. *Biomaterials*, 2014. **35**(1): p. 393–400.

44. West, J.L. and N.J. Halas, Engineered nanomaterials for biophotonics applications: Improving sensing, imaging, and therapeutics. *Annual Review of Biomedical Engineering*, 2003. **5**(1): p. 285–292.

45. Aswathy, R.G., et al., Near-infrared quantum dots for deep tissue imaging. *Analytical and Bioanalytical Chemistry*, 2010. **397**(4): p. 1417–1435.

46. Wang, D., A.L. Rogach, and F. Caruso, Semiconductor quantum dot-labeled microsphere bioconjugates prepared by stepwise self-assembly. *Nano Letters*, 2002. **2**(8): p. 857–861.

47. Md, S., et al., Bromocriptine loaded chitosan nanoparticles intended for direct nose to brain delivery: Pharmacodynamic, pharmacokinetic and scintigraphy study in mice model. *European Journal of Pharmaceutical Sciences*, 2013. **48**(3): p. 393–405.

48. Li, J. and J.-J. Zhu, Quantum dots for fluorescent biosensing and bio-imaging applications. *Analyst*, 2013. **138**(9): p. 2506–2515.

49. Clapp, A.R., I.L. Medintz, and H. Mattoussi, Förster resonance energy transfer investigations using quantum-dot fluorophores. *ChemPhysChem*, 2006. **7**(1): p. 47–57.

50. Roda, A., et al., Nanobioanalytical luminescence: Förster-type energy transfer methods. *Analytical and Bioanalytical Chemistry*, 2009. **393**(1): p. 109–123.

51. Savla, R., et al., Tumor targeted quantum dot-mucin 1 aptamer-doxorubicin conjugate for imaging and treatment of cancer. *Journal of Controlled Release*, 2011. **153**(1): p. 16–22.

52. Jorio, A., G. Dresselhaus, and M.S. Dresselhaus, *Carbon nanotubes: Advanced topics in the synthesis, structure, properties and applications.* Vol. 111. 2007: Springer Science & Business Media.

53. Beguin, F. and P. Ehrburger, *Special issue on carbon nanotubes.* 2002: Pergamon-Elsevier Science Ltd.

54. Ajayan, P.M., Nanotubes from carbon. *Chemical Reviews*, 1999. **99**(7): p. 1787–1800.

55. Wang, J., Carbon-nanotube based electrochemical biosensors: A review. *Electroanalysis: An International Journal Devoted to Fundamental and Practical Aspects of Electroanalysis*, 2005. **17**(1): p. 7–14.

56. Yun, Y., et al., Nanotube electrodes and biosensors. *Nano Today*, 2007. **2**(6): p. 30–37.

57. Kam, N.W.S., et al., Carbon nanotubes as multifunctional biological transporters and near-infrared agents for selective cancer cell destruction. *Proceedings of the National Academy of Sciences*, 2005. **102**(33): p. 11600–11605.

58. Cherukuri, P., et al., Near-infrared fluorescence microscopy of single-walled carbon nanotubes in phagocytic cells. *Journal of the American Chemical Society*, 2004. **126**(48): p. 15638–15639.

59. Lacerda, L., et al., Intracellular trafficking of carbon nanotubes by confocal laser scanning microscopy. *Advanced Materials*, 2007. **19**(11): p. 1480–1484.

60. Singh, R., et al., Tissue biodistribution and blood clearance rates of intravenously administered carbon nanotube radiotracers. *Proceedings of the National Academy of Sciences*, 2006. **103**(9): p. 3357–3362.

61. Riggs, J.E., et al., Strong luminescence of solubilized carbon nanotubes. *Journal of the American Chemical Society*, 2000. **122**(24): p. 5879–5880.

62. Lu, F., et al., Advances in bioapplications of carbon nanotubes. *Advanced Materials*, 2009. **21**(2): p. 139–152.

63. Lin, Y., et al., Visible luminescence of carbon nanotubes and dependence on functionalization. *The Journal of Physical Chemistry B*, 2005. **109**(31): p. 14779–14782.

64. Welsher, K., et al., Selective probing and imaging of cells with single walled carbon nanotubes as near-infrared fluorescent molecules. *Nano Letters*, 2008. **8**(2): p. 586–590.

65. Leeuw, T.K., et al., Single-walled carbon nanotubes in the intact organism: Near-IR imaging and biocompatibility studies in Drosophila. *Nano Letters*, 2007. **7**(9): p. 2650–2654.

66. Nakayama-Ratchford, N., et al., Noncovalent functionalization of carbon nanotubes by fluorescein– polyethylene glycol: Supramolecular conjugates with pH-dependent absorbance and fluorescence. *Journal of the American Chemical Society*, 2007. **129**(9): p. 2448–2449.

67. Porter, A.E., et al., Direct imaging of single-walled carbon nanotubes in cells. *Nature Nanotechnology*, 2007. **2**(11): p. 713–717.

68. Tomalia, D., et al., Reprints of the 1st SPSJ international polymer conference. *The Society of Polymer Science*, 1984. p. 65.

69. Tomalia, D.A., et al., A new class of polymers: Starburst-dendritic macromolecules. *Polymer Journal*, 1985. **17**(1): p. 117–132.

70. Tomalia, D.A., Birth of a new macromolecular architecture: Dendrimers as quantized building blocks for nanoscale synthetic polymer chemistry. *Progress in Polymer Science*, 2005. **30**(3–4): p. 294–324.

71. Tolia, G.T. and H.H. Choi, The role of dendrimers in topical drug delivery. *Pharmaceutical Technology*, 2008. **32**(11): p. 88–98.

72. Madaan, K., et al., Dendrimers in drug delivery and targeting: Drug-dendrimer interactions and toxicity issues. *Journal of Pharmacy & Bioallied Sciences*, 2014. **6**(3): p. 139.

73. Pillai, O. and R. Panchagnula, Polymers in drug delivery. *Current Opinion in Chemical Biology*, 2001. **5**(4): p. 447–451.

74. D'Emanuele, A. and D. Attwood, Dendrimer–drug interactions. *Advanced Drug Delivery Reviews*, 2005. **57**(15): p. 2147–2162.

75. Twibanire, J.-D.A.K. and T.B. Grindley, Efficient and controllably selective preparation of esters using uronium-based coupling agents. *Organic Letters*, 2011. **13**(12): p. 2988–2991.

76. Kolhe, P., et al., Drug complexation, in vitro release and cellular entry of dendrimers and hyperbranched polymers. *International Journal of Pharmaceutics*, 2003. **259**(1–2): p. 143–160.

77. Prajapati, R.N., et al., Dendrimer-mediated solubilization, formulation development and in vitro– in vivo assessment of piroxicam. *Molecular Pharmaceutics*, 2009. **6**(3): p. 940–950.

78. Beezer, A., et al., Dendrimers as potential drug carriers; encapsulation of acidic hydrophobes within water soluble PAMAM derivatives. *Tetrahedron*, 2003. **59**(22): p. 3873–3880.

79. Najlah, M., et al., In vitro evaluation of dendrimer prodrugs for oral drug delivery. *International Journal of Pharmaceutics*, 2007. **336**(1): p. 183–190.

80. Yang, H. and S.T. Lopina, Penicillin V-conjugated PEG-PAMAM star polymers. *Journal of Biomaterials Science, Polymer Edition*, 2003. **14**(10): p. 1043–1056.

81. D'emanuele, A., et al., The use of a dendrimer-propranolol prodrug to bypass efflux transporters and enhance oral bioavailability. *Journal of Controlled Release*, 2004. **95**(3): p. 447–453.

82. Wiener, E., et al., Dendrimer-based metal chelates: A new class of magnetic resonance imaging contrast agents. *Magnetic Resonance in Medicine*, 1994. **31**(1): p. 1–8.

83. Merbach, A.S., L. Helm, and E. Toth, *The chemistry of contrast agents in medical magnetic resonance imaging.* 2013: John Wiley & Sons.

84. Caravan, P., et al., Gadolinium (III) chelates as MRI contrast agents: Structure, dynamics, and applications. *Chemical Reviews*, 1999. **99**(9): p. 2293–2352.

85. Clarkson, R., Blood-pool MRI contrast agents: Properties and characterization. *Contrast Agents I*, 2002: p. 201–235.

86. Langereis, S., et al., Dendrimers and magnetic resonance imaging. *New Journal of Chemistry*, 2007. **31**(7): p. 1152–1160.

87. Dong, Q., et al., Magnetic resonance angiography with gadomer-17: An animal study. *Investigative Radiology*, 1998. **33**(9): p. 699–708.

88. Daldrup-Link, H.E., et al., Comparison of Gadomer-17 and gadopentetate dimeglumine for differentiation of benign from malignant breast tumors with MR imaging. *Academic Radiology*, 2000. **7**(11): p. 934–944.

89. Misselwitz, B., et al., Pharmacokinetics of Gadomer-17, a new dendritic magnetic resonance contrast agent. *Magnetic Resonance Materials in Physics, Biology and Medicine*, 2001. **12**(2–3): p. 128–134.

90. Fink, C., et al., High-resolution three-dimensional MR angiography of rodent tumors: Morphologic characterization of intratumoral vasculature. *Journal of Magnetic Resonance Imaging: An Official Journal of the International Society for Magnetic Resonance in Medicine*, 2003. **18**(1): p. 59–65.

91. Nicolle, G.M., et al., The impact of rigidity and water exchange on the relaxivity of a dendritic MRI contrast agent. *Chemistry–A European Journal*, 2002. **8**(5): p. 1040–1048.

92. Thompson, K.H. and C. Orvig, Boon and bane of metal ions in medicine. *Science*, 2003. **300**(5621): p. 936–939.

93. Choi, Y., et al., DNA-directed synthesis of generation 7 and 5 PAMAM dendrimer nanoclusters. *Nano Letters*, 2004. **4**(3): p. 391–397.

94. van Baal, I., et al., Multivalent peptide and protein dendrimers using native chemical ligation. *Angewandte Chemie*, 2005. **117**(32): p. 5180–5185.

95. Rijkers, D., GW v. Esse, R. Merkx, AJ Brouwer, HJF Jacobs, RJ Pieters, RMJ Liskamp. *Chemical Communications*, 2005. **4581**.

96. Crespo, L., et al., Peptide and amide bond-containing dendrimers. *Chemical Reviews*, 2005. **105**(5): p. 1663–1682.

97. Woller, E.K., et al., Altering the strength of lectin binding interactions and controlling the amount of lectin clustering using mannose/hydroxyl-functionalized dendrimers. *Journal of the American Chemical Society*, 2003. **125**(29): p. 8820–8826.

98. Wolfenden, M.L. and M.J. Cloninger, Mannose/glucose-functionalized dendrimers to investigate the predictable tunability of multivalent interactions. *Journal of the American Chemical Society*, 2005. **127**(35): p. 12168–12169.

99. Zanini, D. and R. Roy, Practical synthesis of starburst PAMAM α-thiosialodendrimers for probing multivalent carbohydrate– lectin binding properties. *The Journal of Organic Chemistry*, 1998. **63**(10): p. 3486–3491.

100. Wu, C., et al., Metal-chelate-dendrimer-antibody constructs for use in radioimmunotherapy and imaging. *Bioorganic & Medicinal Chemistry Letters*, 1994. **4**(3): p. 449–454.

101. Sadler, K. and J.P. Tam, Peptide dendrimers: Applications and synthesis. *Reviews in Molecular Biotechnology*, 2002. **90**(3–4): p. 195–229.

102. Konda, S.D., et al., Development of a tumor-targeting MR contrast agent using the high-affinity folate receptor: Work in progress. *Investigative Radiology*, 2000. **35**(1): p. 50.

103. Konda, S.D., et al., Specific targeting of folate–dendrimer MRI contrast agents to the high affinity folate receptor expressed in ovarian tumor xenografts. *Magnetic Resonance Materials in Physics, Biology and Medicine*, 2001. **12**(2–3): p. 104–113.

104. Konda, S.D., et al., Biodistribution of a 153Gd-folate dendrimer, generation= 4, in mice with folate-receptor positive and negative ovarian tumor xenografts. *Investigative Radiology*, 2002. **37**(4): p. 199–204.

105. Barrett, T., et al., Dendrimers application related to bioimaging. *IEEE Engineering in Medicine and Biology Magazine: The Quarterly Magazine of the Engineering in Medicine & Biology Society*, 2009. **28**(1): p. 12.

106. Bielinska, A., et al., Imaging {Au 0-PAMAM} gold-dendrimer nanocomposites in cells. *Journal of Nanoparticle Research*, 2002. **4**(5): p. 395–403.

107. Levingstone, T.J., S. Herbaj, and N.J. Dunne, Calcium phosphate nanoparticles for therapeutic applications in bone regeneration. *Nanomaterials*, 2019. **9**(11): p. 1570.

108. Sokolova, V.V., et al., Effective transfection of cells with multi-shell calcium phosphate-DNA nanoparticles. *Biomaterials*, 2006. **27**(16): p. 3147–3153.

109. Cai, Y. and R. Tang, Calcium phosphate nanoparticles in biomineralization and biomaterials. *Journal of Materials Chemistry*, 2008. **18**(32): p. 3775–3787.

110. Maitra, A., Calcium phosphate nanoparticles: Second-generation nonviral vectors in gene therapy. *Expert Review of Molecular Diagnostics*, 2005. **5**(6): p. 893–905.

111. Epple, M., et al., Application of calcium phosphate nanoparticles in biomedicine. *Journal of Materials Chemistry*, 2010. **20**(1): p. 18–23.

112. Altınoğ˘lu, E.I., et al., Near-infrared emitting fluorophore-doped calcium phosphate nanoparticles for in vivo imaging of human breast cancer. *ACS Nano*, 2008. **2**(10): p. 2075–2084.

113. Zhou, Z.-X., et al., Drug packaging and delivery using perfluorocarbon nanoparticles for targeted inhibition of vascular smooth muscle cells. *Acta Pharmacologica Sinica*, 2009. **30**(11): p. 1577–1584.

114. Tran, T.D., et al., Clinical applications of perfluorocarbon nanoparticles for molecular imaging and targeted therapeutics. *International Journal of Nanomedicine*, 2007. **2**(4): p. 515.

115. Winter, P.M., et al., Emerging nanomedicine opportunities with perfluorocarbon nanoparticles. *Expert Review of Medical Devices*, 2007. **4**(2): p. 137–145.

116. Noveck, R.J., et al., Randomized safety studies of intravenous perflubron emulsion. II. Effects on immune function in healthy volunteers. *Anesthesia & Analgesia*, 2000. **91**(4): p. 812–822.

117. Leese, P.T., et al., Randomized safety studies of intravenous perflubron emulsion. I. Effects on coagulation function in healthy volunteers. *Anesthesia & Analgesia*, 2000. **91**(4): p. 804–811.

118. Fan, X., et al., MRI of perfluorocarbon emulsion kinetics in rodent mammary tumours. *Physics in Medicine & Biology*, 2005. **51**(2): p. 211.

119. Partlow, K.C., et al., 19F magnetic resonance imaging for stem/progenitor cell tracking with multiple unique perfluorocarbon nanobeacons. *The FASEB Journal*, 2007. **21**(8): p. 1647–1654.

120. Koshkina, O., et al., Multicore liquid perfluorocarbon-loaded multimodal nanoparticles for stable ultrasound and 19F MRI applied to In vivo cell tracking. *Advanced Functional Materials*, 2019. **29**(19): p. 1806485.

121. DiStasio, N., et al., The multifaceted uses and therapeutic advantages of nanoparticles for atherosclerosis research. *Materials*, 2018. **11**(5): p. 754.

122. Dang, J., et al., Manipulating tumor hypoxia toward enhanced photodynamic therapy (PDT). *Biomaterials Science*, 2017. **5**(8): p. 1500–1511.

123. Winter, P., et al., Improved paramagnetic chelate for molecular imaging with MRI. *Journal of Magnetism and Magnetic Materials*, 2005. **293**(1): p. 540–545.

124. Lanza, G.M., et al., A novel site-targeted ultrasonic contrast agent with broad biomedical application. *Circulation*, 1996. **94**(12): p. 3334–3340.

125. Xu, X., et al., Microfluidic production of nanoscale perfluorocarbon droplets as liquid contrast agents for ultrasound imaging. *Lab on a Chip*, 2017. **17**(20): p. 3504–3513.

126. Lijowski, M., et al., High-resolution SPECT-CT/MR molecular imaging of angiogenesis in the Vx2 model. *Investigative Radiology*, 2009. **44**(1): p. 15.

127. Chen, J., et al., Perfluorocarbon nanoparticles for physiological and molecular imaging and therapy. *Advances in Chronic Kidney Disease*, 2013. **20**(6): p. 466–478.

128. Verma, A. and A. Verma, Polyelectrolyte complex-an overview. *International Journal of Pharmaceutical Sciences and Research*, 2013. **4**(5): p. 1684.

129. Zare, E.N., et al., Metal-based nanostructures/PLGA nanocomposites: Antimicrobial activity, cytotoxicity, and their biomedical applications. *ACS Applied Materials & Interfaces*, 2019. **12**(3): p. 3279–3300.

130. Taber, L. and A. Umerska, Polyelectrolyte complexes as nanoparticulate drug delivery systems. *European Pharmaceutical Review*, 2015. **20**(3): p. 36–40.

131. Joye, I.J. and D.J. McClements, Biopolymer-based nanoparticles and microparticles: Fabrication, characterization, and application. *Current Opinion in Colloid & Interface Science*, 2014. **19**(5): p. 417–427.

132. Meka, V.S., et al., A comprehensive review on polyelectrolyte complexes. *Drug Discovery Today*, 2017. **22**(11): p. 1697–1706.

133. Dul, M., et al., Self-assembled carrageenan/protamine polyelectrolyte nanoplexes— Investigation of critical parameters governing their formation and characteristics. *Carbohydrate Polymers*, 2015. **123**: p. 339–349.

134. Montero, N., et al., Development of polyelectrolyte complex nanoparticles-PECNs loaded with ampicillin by means of polyelectrolyte complexation and ultra-high pressure homogenization (UHPH). *Polymers*, 2020. **12**(5): p. 1168.

135. Ferjaoui, Z., et al., Layer-by-layer self-assembly of polyelectrolytes on superparamagnetic nanoparticle surfaces. *ACS Omega*, 2020. **5**(10): p. 4770–4777.

136. Hugerth, A., N. Caram-Lelham, and L.-O. Sundelöf, The effect of charge density and conformation on the polyelectrolyte complex formation between carrageenan and chitosan. *Carbohydrate Polymers*, 1997. **34**(3): p. 149–156.

137. Ramasamy, T., et al., Chitosan-based polyelectrolyte complexes as potential nanoparticulate carriers: Physicochemical and biological characterization. *Pharmaceutical Research*, 2014. **31**(5): p. 1302–1314.

138. Amani, S., Z. Mohamadnia, and A. Mahdavi, pH-responsive hybrid magnetic polyelectrolyte complex based on alginate/BSA as efficient nanocarrier for curcumin encapsulation and delivery. *International Journal of Biological Macromolecules*, 2019. **141**: p. 1258–1270.

139. Zhan, R. and B. Liu, Benzothiadiazole-containing conjugated polyelectrolytes for biological sensing and imaging. *Macromolecular Chemistry and Physics*, 2015. **216**(2): p. 131–144.

140. Feng, G., J. Liang, and B. Liu, Hyperbranched conjugated polyelectrolytes for biological sensing and imaging. *Macromolecular Rapid Communications*, 2013. **34**(9): p. 705–715.

141. Zahraei, M., et al., Synthesis and characterization of chitosan coated manganese zinc ferrite nanoparticles as MRI contrast agents. *Journal of Nanostructures*, 2015. **5**(2): p. 77–86.

142. Hartig, S.M., et al., Multifunctional nanoparticulate polyelectrolyte complexes. *Pharmaceutical Research*, 2007. **24**(12): p. 2353–2369.

143. Hesselink, J.R., R.R. Edelman, and M. Zlatkin, *Clinical magnetic resonance imaging*. 1990: Saunders.

144. Schenck, J.F., The role of magnetic susceptibility in magnetic resonance imaging: MRI magnetic compatibility of the first and second kinds. *Medical Physics*, 1996. **23**(6): p. 815–850.

145. Ghaghada, K.B., et al., Pre-clinical evaluation of a nanoparticle-based blood-pool contrast agent for MR imaging of the placenta. *Placenta*, 2017. **57**: p. 60–70.

146. Padmanabhan, P., et al., Nanoparticles in practice for molecular-imaging applications: An overview. *Acta Biomaterialia*, 2016. **41**: p. 1–16.

147. Sedivy, P., et al., 31P-MR spectroscopy in patients with mild and serious lower limb ischemia. *International Angiology: A Journal of the International Union of Angiology*, 2018. **37**(4): p. 293.

148. Suzuki, K., et al., Ligand-based molecular MRI: O-17 JJVCPE amyloid imaging in transgenic mice. *Journal of Neuroimaging*, 2014. **24**(6): p. 595–598.

149. Srinivas, M., et al., Labeling cells for in vivo tracking using 19F MRI. *Biomaterials*, 2012. **33**(34): p. 8830–8840.

150. Gonzales, C., et al., In-vivo detection and tracking of T cells in various organs in a melanoma tumor model by 19F-fluorine MRS/MRI. *PloS One*, 2016. **11**(10): p. e0164557.

151. Arbab, A.S., et al., A model of lysosomal metabolism of dextran coated superparamagnetic iron oxide (SPIO) nanoparticles: Implications for cellular magnetic resonance imaging. *NMR in Biomedicine: An International Journal Devoted to the Development and Application of Magnetic Resonance In Vivo*, 2005. **18**(6): p. 383–389.

152. Laus, S., et al., Rotational dynamics account for pH-dependent relaxivities of PAMAM dendrimeric, Gd-based potential MRI contrast agents. *Chemistry–A European Journal*, 2005. **11**(10): p. 3064–3076.

153. Knight, J.C., P.G. Edwards, and S.J. Paisey, Fluorinated contrast agents for magnetic resonance imaging; a review of recent developments. *RSC Advances*, 2011. **1**(8): p. 1415–1425.

154. Saito, R., et al., Gadolinium-loaded liposomes allow for real-time magnetic resonance imaging of convection-enhanced delivery in the primate brain. *Experimental Neurology*, 2005. **196**(2): p. 381–389.

155. Buzug, T.M., Computed tomography. In Kramme R., Hoffmann KP., Pozos R.S. (eds) *Springer handbook of medical technology.* 2011: Springer Handbooks. Springer. p. 311–342.

156. Pelc, N.J., Recent and future directions in CT imaging. *Annals of Biomedical Engineering*, 2014. **42**(2): p. 260–268.

157. Ghaghada, K.B., et al., Computed tomography imaging of solid tumors using a liposomal-iodine contrast agent in companion dogs with naturally occurring cancer. *PloS One*, 2016. **11**(3): p. e0152718.

158. Fenster, A., D.B. Downey, and H.N. Cardinal, Three-dimensional ultrasound imaging. *Physics in Medicine & Biology*, 2001. **46**(5): p. R67.

159. Szabo, T.L., *Diagnostic ultrasound imaging: Inside out.* 2004: Academic Press.

160. Terris, M.K. and T.A. Stamey, Determination of prostate volume by transrectal ultrasound. *The Journal of Urology*, 1991. **145**(5): p. 984–987.

161. Rösch, T., et al., Endoscopic ultrasound in pancreatic tumor diagnosis. *Gastrointestinal Endoscopy*, 1991. **37**(3): p. 347–352.

162. Maisey, M.N., Positron emission tomography in clinical medicine, in Peter E. Valk, Dominique Delbeke, Dale L. Bailey, David W. Townsend, and Michael N. Maisey (Eds) *Positron emission tomography.* 2005: Springer. p. 1–12.

163. Berger, A., How does it work?: Positron emission tomography. *BMJ: British Medical Journal*, 2003. **326**(7404): p. 1449.

164. National Research Council, Single photon emission computed tomography, in *Mathematics and physics of emerging biomedical imaging.* 1996: Washington (DC) National Academies Press (US) and Institute of Medicine (US) Committee on the Mathematics and Physics of Emerging Dynamic Biomedical Imaging.

165. Madru, R., et al., 99mTc-labeled superparamagnetic iron oxide nanoparticles for multimodality SPECT/MRI of sentinel lymph nodes. *Journal of Nuclear Medicine*, 2012. **53**(3): p. 459–463.

166. Bouziotis, P., et al., Radiolabeled iron oxide nanoparticles as dual-modality SPECT/MRI and PET/MRI agents. *Current Topics in Medicinal Chemistry*, 2012. **12**(23): p. 2694–2702.

167. Buck, A.K., et al., Spect/ct. *Journal of Nuclear Medicine*, 2008. **49**(8): p. 1305–1319.

168. Zhao, L., et al., Chlorotoxin peptide-functionalized polyethylenimine-entrapped gold nanoparticles for glioma SPECT/CT imaging and radionuclide therapy. *Journal of Nanobiotechnology*, 2019. **17**(1): p. 30.

169. Tseng, Y.-C., et al., Lipid–calcium phosphate nanoparticles for delivery to the lymphatic system and SPECT/CT imaging of lymph node metastases. *Biomaterials*, 2014. **35**(16): p. 4688–4698.

170. Chrastina, A. and J.E. Schnitzer, Iodine-125 radiolabeling of silver nanoparticles for in vivo SPECT imaging. *International Journal of Nanomedicine*, 2010. **5**: p. 653.

171. Qi, H., et al., Biomass-derived nitrogen-doped carbon quantum dots: Highly selective fluorescent probe for detecting Fe^{3+} ions and tetracyclines. *Journal of Colloid and Interface Science*, 2019. **539**: p. 332–341.

172. Miyawaki, A., Fluorescence imaging of physiological activity in complex systems using GFP-based probes. *Current Opinion in Neurobiology*, 2003. **13**(5): p. 591–596.

173. Kapuscinski, J., DAPI: A DNA-specific fluorescent probe. *Biotechnic & Histochemistry*, 1995. **70**(5): p. 220–233.

174. Yin, J., et al., Cyanine-based fluorescent probe for highly selective detection of glutathione in cell cultures and live mouse tissues. *Journal of the American Chemical Society*, 2014. **136**(14): p. 5351–5358.

175. Wang, X., et al., Screening and investigation of a cyanine fluorescent probe for simultaneous sensing of glutathione and cysteine under single excitation. *Chemical Communications*, 2014. **50**(97): p. 15439–15442.

176. Pleijhuis, R., et al., Near-infrared fluorescence (NIRF) imaging in breast-conserving surgery: Assessing intraoperative techniques in tissue-simulating breast phantoms. *European Journal of Surgical Oncology (EJSO)*, 2011. **37**(1): p. 32–39.

177. Luker, G.D. and K.E. Luker, Optical imaging: Current applications and future directions. *Journal of Nuclear Medicine*, 2008. **49**(1): p. 1–4.

178. Daldrup-Link, H.E., et al., Cell tracking with gadophrin-2: a bifunctional contrast agent for MR imaging, optical imaging, and fluorescence microscopy. *European Journal of Nuclear Medicine and Molecular Imaging*, 2004. **31**(9): p. 1312–1321.

179. Pillarisetti, S., et al., Multimodal composite iron oxide nanoparticles for biomedical applications. *Tissue Engineering and Regenerative Medicine*, 2019: **16**: p. 451–465.

180. Lee, M.J.-E., et al., Rapid pharmacokinetic and biodistribution studies using cholorotoxin-conjugated iron oxide nanoparticles: a novel non-radioactive method. *PloS One*, 2010. **5**(3): p. e9536.

181. Leung, K., *HiLyte Fluor 647-hyaluronic acid-gold nanoparticles*. 2009: europe PMC.

182. Lee, D.-E., et al., Hyaluronidase-sensitive SPIONs for MR/optical dual imaging nanoprobes. *Macromolecular Research*, 2011. **19**(8): p. 861–867.

183. Yang, L., et al., uPAR-targeted optical imaging contrasts as theranostic agents for tumor margin detection. *Theranostics*, 2014. **4**(1): p. 106.

184. Peng, H., et al., DNA hybridization detection with blue luminescent quantum dots and dye-labeled single-stranded DNA. *Journal of the American Chemical Society*, 2007. **129**(11): p. 3048–3049.

185. Gill, R., et al., Fluorescence resonance energy transfer in CdSe/ZnS– DNA conjugates: Probing hybridization and DNA cleavage. *The Journal of Physical Chemistry B*, 2005. **109**(49): p. 23715–23719.

186. Edgar, R., et al., High-sensitivity bacterial detection using biotin-tagged phage and quantum-dot nanocomplexes. *Proceedings of the National Academy of Sciences*, 2006. **103**(13): p. 4841–4845.

187. Goldman, E.R., et al., Multiplexed toxin analysis using four colors of quantum dot fluororeagents. *Analytical Chemistry*, 2004. **76**(3): p. 684–688.

188. Haschek, W.M., C.G. Rousseaux, and M.A. Wallig, *Haschek and Rousseaux's handbook of toxicologic pathology*. 2013: Academic Press.

189. Xu, M. and L.V. Wang, Photoacoustic imaging in biomedicine. *Review of Scientific Instruments*, 2006. **77**(4): p. 041101.

190. Weber, J., P.C. Beard, and S.E. Bohndiek, Contrast agents for molecular photoacoustic imaging. *Nature Methods*, 2016. **13**(8): p. 639–650.

191. Yang, X., et al., Nanoparticles for photoacoustic imaging. *Wiley Interdisciplinary Reviews: Nanomedicine and Nanobiotechnology*, 2009. **1**(4): p. 360–368.

192. Dai, Y., et al., Nanoparticle design strategies for enhanced anticancer therapy by exploiting the tumour microenvironment. *Chemical Society Reviews*, 2017. **46**(12): p. 3830–3852.

193. De La Zerda, A., et al., Carbon nanotubes as photoacoustic molecular imaging agents in living mice. *Nature Nanotechnology*, 2008. **3**(9): p. 557–562.

194. Zhou, G., et al., Porphyrin–palladium hydride MOF nanoparticles for tumor-targeting photoacoustic imaging-guided hydrogenothermal cancer therapy. *Nanoscale Horizons*, 2019. **4**(5): p. 1185–1193.

195. Wang, C., et al., RGD-conjugated silica-coated gold nanorods on the surface of carbon nanotubes for targeted photoacoustic imaging of gastric cancer. *Nanoscale Research Letters*, 2014. **9**(1): p. 1–10.

196. Ustione, A. and D. Piston, A simple introduction to multiphoton microscopy. *Journal of Microscopy*, 2011. **243**(3): p. 221–226.

197. Williams, R.M., W.R. Zipfel, and W.W. Webb, Multiphoton microscopy in biological research. *Current Opinion in Chemical Biology*, 2001. **5**(5): p. 603–608.

198. Christie, R., et al., Growth arrest of individual senile plaques in a model of Alzheimer's disease observed by in vivo multiphoton microscopy. *Journal of Neuroscience*, 2001. **21**(3): p. 858–864.

199. Tozer, G.M., et al., Intravital imaging of tumour vascular networks using multi-photon fluorescence microscopy. *Advanced Drug Delivery Reviews*, 2005. **57**(1): p. 135–152.

200. Frolov, A., et al., High density lipoprotein-mediated cholesterol uptake and targeting to lipid droplets in intact L-cell fibroblasts A single-and multiphoton fluorescence approach. *Journal of Biological Chemistry*, 2000. **275**(17): p. 12769–12780.

201. Kleinhans, C., K.W. Kafitz, and C.R. Rose, Multi-photon intracellular sodium imaging combined with UV-mediated focal uncaging of glutamate in CA1 pyramidal neurons. *JoVE (Journal of Visualized Experiments)*, 2014. 92: p. e52038.

202. Engert, F. and T. Bonhoeffer, Dendritic spine changes associated with hippocampal long-term synaptic plasticity. *Nature*, 1999. **399**(6731): p. 66–70.

203. Boksebeld, M., et al., Folate-modified silicon carbide nanoparticles as multiphoton imaging nanoprobes for cancer-cell-specific labeling. *RSC Advances*, 2017. **7**(44): p. 27361–27369.

204. Lakowicz, J.R., et al., Emission spectral properties of cadmium sulfide nanoparticles with multiphoton excitation. *The Journal of Physical Chemistry B*, 2002. **106**(21): p. 5365–5370.

205. Dowling, M.B., et al., Multiphoton-absorption-induced-luminescence (MAIL) imaging of tumor-targeted gold nanoparticles. *Bioconjugate Chemistry*, 2010. **21**(11): p. 1968–1977.

206. Day, E.S., et al., Antibody-conjugated gold-gold sulfide nanoparticles as multifunctional agents for imaging and therapy of breast cancer. *International Journal of Nanomedicine*, 2010. **5**: p. 445.

207. Rahim, N.A.A., et al., Conjugated polymer nanoparticles for two-photon imaging of endothelial cells in a tissue model. *Advanced Materials*, 2009. **21**(34): p. 3492–3496.

208. Nakashima, J. and H. Duong, *Radiology, image production and evaluation*. 2020.

209. Gerber, S., et al., Imaging of sacral tumours. *Skeletal Radiology*, 2008. **37**(4): p. 277–289.

210. Egan, R.L., *Breast imaging: Diagnosis and morphology of breast diseases*. 1988: INIS.IAEA.

211. Katz, D.S. and A.N. Leung, Radiology of pneumonia. *Clinics in Chest Medicine*, 1999. **20**(3): p. 549–562.

212. Rastogi, A.K., et al., Fundamentals of joint injection. *American Journal of Roentgenology*, 2016. **207**(3): p. 484–494.

213. Cwikiel, W., et al., Malignant esophageal strictures: Treatment with a self-expanding nitinol stent. *Radiology*, 1993. **187**(3): p. 661–665.

214. Jackson, P., et al., Evaluation of the effects of gold nanoparticle shape and size on contrast enhancement in radiological imaging. *Australasian Physical & Engineering Sciences in Medicine*, 2011. **34**(2): p. 243.

215. Cole, L.E., et al., Gold nanoparticles as contrast agents in x-ray imaging and computed tomography. *Nanomedicine*, 2015. **10**(2): p. 321–341.

216. Lee, Y.K., et al., Novel method of producing nanoparticles for gadolinium-scintillator-based digital radiography. *Journal of Nanoscience and Nanotechnology*, 2013. **13**(10): p. 7026–7029.

217. Thrall, J.H., J.E. Freitas, and W.H. Beierwaltes (eds). Adrenal scintigraphy, in *Seminars in nuclear medicine*. 1978: Elsevier.

218. Gross, M.D., et al., Contemporary adrenal scintigraphy. European Journal of Nuclear Medicine and Molecular Imaging, 2007. **34**(4): p. 547–557.

219. Majd, M. and H.G. Rushton (eds). Renal cortical scintigraphy in the diagnosis of acute pyelonephritis, in *Seminars in nuclear medicine*. 1992: Elsevier.

220. Kotler, T.S. and G.A. Diamond, Exercise thallium-201 scintigraphy in the diagnosis and prognosis of coronary artery disease. *Annals of Internal Medicine*, 1990. **113**(9): p. 684–702.

221. Nagayama, H., et al., Reliability of MIBG myocardial scintigraphy in the diagnosis of Parkinson's disease. *Journal of Neurology, Neurosurgery & Psychiatry*, 2005. **76**(2): p. 249–251.

222. McDougall, I.R., Skeletal scintigraphy. *Western Journal of Medicine*, 1979. **130**(6): p. 503.

223. Fitzgerald, P., et al., A γ-scintigraphic evaluation of microparticulate ophthalmic delivery systems: Liposomes and nanoparticles. *International Journal of Pharmaceutics*, 1987. **40**(1–2): p. 81–84.

224. Khan, A., et al., Brain targeting of temozolomide via the intranasal route using lipid-based nanoparticles: Brain pharmacokinetic and scintigraphic analyses. *Molecular Pharmaceutics*, 2016. **13**(11): p. 3773–3782.

225. Alric, C., et al., The biodistribution of gold nanoparticles designed for renal clearance. *Nanoscale*, 2013. **5**(13): p. 5930–5939.

226. Raj, P.M., et al., Biodistribution and targeting potential assessment of mucoadhesive chitosan nanoparticles designed for ulcerative colitis via scintigraphy. *RSC Advances*, 2018. **8**(37): p. 20809–20821.

227. Ayan, A.K., A. Yenilmez, and H. Eroglu, Evaluation of radiolabeled curcumin-loaded solid lipid nanoparticles usage as an imaging agent in liver-spleen scintigraphy. *Materials Science and Engineering: C*, 2017. **75**: p. 663–670.

228. Chauhan, R.P., et al., Evaluation of folate conjugated superparamagnetic iron oxide nanoparticles for scintigraphic/magnetic resonance imaging. *Journal of Biomedical Nanotechnology*, 2013. **9**(3): p. 323–334.

229. Imam, S.S., et al., Formulation and optimization of levofloxacin loaded chitosan nanoparticle for ocular delivery: In-vitro characterization, ocular tolerance and antibacterial activity. *International Journal of Biological Macromolecules*, 2018. **108**: p. 650–659.

230. Katiyar, S., et al., In situ gelling dorzolamide loaded chitosan nanoparticles for the treatment of glaucoma. *Carbohydrate Polymers*, 2014. **102**: p. 117–124.

231. Jafarieh, O., et al., Design, characterization, and evaluation of intranasal delivery of ropinirole-loaded mucoadhesive nanoparticles for brain targeting. *Drug Development and Industrial Pharmacy*, 2015. **41**(10): p. 1674–1681.

232. Elnaggar, Y.S., et al., Intranasal piperine-loaded chitosan nanoparticles as brain-targeted therapy in Alzheimer's disease: Optimization, biological efficacy, and potential toxicity. *Journal of Pharmaceutical Sciences*, 2015. **104**(10): p. 3544–3556.

233. Kircher, M.F., S.S. Gambhir, and J. Grimm, Noninvasive cell-tracking methods. *Nature Reviews Clinical Oncology*, 2011. **8**(11): p. 677.

234. Alam, S.R., et al., Ultrasmall superparamagnetic particles of iron oxide in patients with acute myocardial infarction: Early clinical experience. *Circulation: Cardiovascular Imaging*, 2012. **5**(5): p. 559–565.

235. Sosnovik, D.E. and M. Nahrendorf, Cells and iron oxide nanoparticles on the move: Magnetic resonance imaging of monocyte homing and myocardial inflammation in patients with ST-elevation myocardial infarction. *Circulation: Cardiovascular Imaging*, 2012. **5**(5): p. 551–554.

236. Kircher, M.F., et al., In vivo high resolution three-dimensional imaging of antigen-specific cytotoxic T-lymphocyte trafficking to tumors. *Cancer Research*, 2003. **63**(20): p. 6838–6846.

237. Pittet, M.J., et al., In vivo imaging of T cell delivery to tumors after adoptive transfer therapy. *Proceedings of the National Academy of Sciences*, 2007. **104**(30): p. 12457–12461.

238. Zhou, R., et al., In vivo detection of stem cells grafted in infarcted rat myocardium. *Journal of Nuclear Medicine*, 2005. **46**(5): p. 816–822.

239. Grimm, J., et al., A nanoparticle-based cell labeling agent for cell tracking with SPECT/CT. *Mol Imaging*, 2006. **5**(Suppl 3): p. 364.

240. Astolfo, A., et al., In vivo visualization of gold-loaded cells in mice using x-ray computed tomography. *Nanomedicine: Nanotechnology, Biology and Medicine*, 2013. **9**(2): p. 284–292.

241. Gilad, A.A., et al., MR tracking of transplanted cells with "positive contrast" using manganese oxide nanoparticles. *Magnetic Resonance in Medicine: An Official Journal of the International Society for Magnetic Resonance in Medicine*, 2008. **60**(1): p. 1–7.

242. Pala, A., et al., Labelling of granulocytes by phagocytic engulfment with 64 Cu-labelled chitosan-coated magnetic nanoparticles. *Molecular Imaging and Biology*, 2012. **14**(5): p. 593–598.

243. Zhu, J., L. Zhou, and F. XingWu, Tracking neural stem cells in patients with brain trauma. *New England Journal of Medicine*, 2006. **355**(22): p. 2376–2378.

244. Leike, J., A. Sachse, and C. Ehritt, Biodistribution and CT-imaging characteristics of iopromide-carrying liposomes in rats. *Journal of Liposome Research*, 1996. **6**(4): p. 665–680.

245. Krause, W., et al., Characterization of iopromide liposomes. *Investigative Radiology*, 1993. **28**(11): p. 1028–1032.

246. Hallouard, F., et al., Iodinated blood pool contrast media for preclinical X-ray imaging applications–A review. *Biomaterials*, 2010. **31**(24): p. 6249–6268.

247. de Vries, A., et al., Block-copolymer-stabilized iodinated emulsions for use as CT contrast agents. *Biomaterials*, 2010. **31**(25): p. 6537–6544.

248. Torchilin, V.P., M.D. Frank-Kamenetsky, and G.L. Wolf, CT visualization of blood pool in rats by using long-circulating, iodine-containing micelles. *Academic Radiology*, 1999. **6**(1): p. 61–65.

249. Kong, W.H., et al., Nanoparticulate carrier containing water-insoluble iodinated oil as a multifunctional contrast agent for computed tomography imaging. *Biomaterials*, 2007. **28**(36): p. 5555–5561.

250. Aviv, H., et al., Radiopaque iodinated copolymeric nanoparticles for X-ray imaging applications. *Biomaterials*, 2009. **30**(29): p. 5610–5616.

251. Liu, Y., Hybrid BaYbF 5 nanoparticles: Novel binary contrast agent for high-resolution in vivo X-ray computed tomography angiography, in *Multifunctional nanoprobes*. Springer Theses (Recognizing Outstanding Ph.D. Research) 2018: Springer. p. 105–120.

252. Weissleder, R., et al., The diagnosis of splenic lymphoma by MR imaging: Value of superparamagnetic iron oxide. *American Journal of Roentgenology*, 1989. **152**(1): p. 175–180.

253. Kim, Y.K., et al., Hepatocellular carcinoma in patients with chronic liver disease: Comparison of SPIO-enhanced MR imaging and 16–detector row CT. *Radiology*, 2006. **238**(2): p. 531–541.

254. Mack, M.G., et al., Superparamagnetic iron oxide–enhanced MR imaging of head and neck lymph nodes. *Radiology*, 2002. **222**(1): p. 239–244.

255. Schmitz, S.A., et al., Magnetic resonance imaging of atherosclerotic plaques using superparamagnetic iron oxide particles. *Journal of Magnetic Resonance Imaging: An Official Journal of the International Society for Magnetic Resonance in Medicine*, 2001. **14**(4): p. 355–361.

256. Harisinghani, M.G., et al., Noninvasive detection of clinically occult lymph-node metastases in prostate cancer. *New England Journal of Medicine*, 2003. **348**(25): p. 2491–2499.

257. Saleh, A., et al., Central nervous system inflammatory response after cerebral infarction as detected by magnetic resonance imaging. *NMR in Biomedicine: An International Journal Devoted to the Development and Application of Magnetic Resonance In Vivo*, 2004. **17**(4): p. 163–169.

258. Kim, S., et al., Near-infrared fluorescent type II quantum dots for sentinel lymph node mapping. *Nature Biotechnology*, 2004. **22**(1): p. 93–97.

259. Cai, X., et al., In vivo quantitative evaluation of the transport kinetics of gold nanocages in a lymphatic system by noninvasive photoacoustic tomography. *ACS Nano*, 2011. **5**(12): p. 9658–9667.

260. Ocampo-García, B.E., et al., 99mTc-labelled gold nanoparticles capped with HYNIC-peptide/mannose for sentinel lymph node detection. *Nuclear Medicine and Biology*, 2011. **38**(1): p. 1–11.

261. Sever, A.R., et al., Preoperative needle biopsy of sentinel lymph nodes using intradermal microbubbles and contrast-enhanced ultrasound in patients with breast cancer. *American Journal of Roentgenology*, 2012. **199**(2): p. 465–470.

262. Weissleder, R., Liver MR imaging with iron oxides: Toward consensus and clinical practice. *Radiology*, 1994. **193**(3): p. 593–595.

263. Rappeport, E., et al., Contrast-enhanced FDG-PET/CT vs. SPIO-enhanced MRI vs. FDG-PET vs. CT in patients with liver metastases from colorectal cancer: a prospective study with intraoperative confirmation. *Acta Radiologica*, 2007. **48**(4): p. 369–378.

264. Ward, J., et al., Colorectal hepatic metastases: Detection with SPIO-enhanced breath-hold MR imaging—Comparison of optimized sequences. *Radiology*, 2003. **228**(3): p. 709–718.

265. Yamamoto, H., et al., MR enhancement of hepatoma by superparamagnetic iron oxide (SPIO) particles. *Journal of Computer Assisted Tomography*, 1995. **19**(4): p. 665–667.

266. Denis, M.C., et al., Imaging inflammation of the pancreatic islets in type 1 diabetes. *Proceedings of the National Academy of Sciences*, 2004. **101**(34): p. 12634–12639.

267. Gaglia, J.L., et al., Noninvasive imaging of pancreatic islet inflammation in type 1A diabetes patients. *The Journal of Clinical Investigation*, 2011. **121**(1): p. 442–445.

268. Wang, X., et al., Au-nanoparticle coated mesoporous silica nanocapsule-based multifunctional platform for ultrasound mediated imaging, cytoclasis and tumor ablation. *Biomaterials*, 2013. **34**(8): p. 2057–2068.

269. Niu, D., et al., Facile synthesis of magnetite/perfluorocarbon co-loaded organic/inorganic hybrid vesicles for dual-modality ultrasound/magnetic resonance imaging and imaging-guided high-intensity focused ultrasound ablation. *Advanced Materials*, 2013. **25**(19): p. 2686–2692.

270. Maier-Hauff, K., et al., Efficacy and safety of intratumoral thermotherapy using magnetic iron-oxide nanoparticles combined with external beam radiotherapy on patients with recurrent glioblastoma multiforme. *Journal of Neuro-Oncology*, 2011. **103**(2): p. 317–324.

271. Xu, Q.C., et al., Anti-cAngptl4 Ab-conjugated N–TiO2/NaYF4: Yb, Tm nanocomposite for near infrared-triggered drug release and enhanced targeted cancer cell ablation. *Advanced Healthcare Materials*, 2012. **1**(4): p. 470–474.

272. Shen, H., et al., Cooperative, nanoparticle-enabled thermal therapy of breast cancer. *Advanced Healthcare Materials*, 2012. **1**(1): p. 84–89.

273. Su, Y., et al., Gold nanoparticles-decorated silicon nanowires as highly efficient near-infrared hyperthermia agents for cancer cells destruction. *Nano Letters*, 2012. **12**(4): p. 1845–1850.

274. Lammers, T., et al., Nanotheranostics and image-guided drug delivery: Current concepts and future directions. *Molecular Pharmaceutics*, 2010. **7**(6): p. 1899–1912.

275. Minchin, R.F. and D.J. Martin, Minireview: Nanoparticles for molecular imaging—An overview. *Endocrinology*, 2010. **151**(2): p. 474–481.

276. Zhang, W.L., et al., Gadolinium-conjugated folate–poly (ethylene glycol)–polyamidoamine dendrimer–carboxyl nanoparticles as potential tumor-targeted, circulation-prolonged macromolecular magnetic resonance imaging contrast agents. II. *Journal of Applied Polymer Science*, 2011. **121**(6): p. 3175–3184.

277. van Kasteren, S.I., et al., Glyconanoparticles allow pre-symptomatic in vivo imaging of brain disease. *Proceedings of the National Academy of Sciences*, 2009. **106**(1): p. 18–23.

278. Veiseh, O., et al., Optical and MRI multifunctional nanoprobe for targeting gliomas. *Nano Letters*, 2005. **5**(6): p. 1003–1008.

279. Gambhir, S., et al., Imaging transgene expression with radionuclide imaging technologies. *Neoplasia*, 2000. **2**(1–2): p. 118–138.

280. Law, B. and C.-H. Tung, 7.3 Fluorescence reporters for biomedical imaging, in *Textbook of in vivo imaging in vertebrates*, 2007: p. 203.

281. Sun, C., et al., *Tumor-targeted drug delivery and MRI contrast enhancement by chlorotoxin-conjugated iron oxide nanoparticles*, Future Medicine 2008.

282. Juríková, A., et al., Thermal analysis of magnetic nanoparticles modified with dextran. *Acta Physica Polonica-Series A General Physics*, 2012. **121**(5): p. 1296.

283. Akgun, H., et al., Are gadolinium-based contrast media nephrotoxic?: A renal biopsy study. *Archives of Pathology & Laboratory Medicine*, 2006. **130**(9): p. 1354–1357.

284. Thomsen, H.S., Gadolinium-based contrast media may be nephrotoxic even at approved doses. *European Radiology*, 2004. **14**(9): p. 1654–1656.

285. Lee, K., et al., Optical imaging of intracellular reactive oxygen species for the assessment of the cytotoxicity of nanoparticles. *Biomaterials*, 2011. **32**(10): p. 2556–2565.

286. Lewinski, N., V. Colvin, and R. Drezek, Cytotoxicity of nanoparticles. *Small*, 2008. **4**(1): p. 26–49.

287. Dong, X., et al., In vivo imaging tracking and immune responses to nanovaccines involving combined antigen nanoparticles with a programmed delivery. *ACS Applied Materials & Interfaces*, 2018. **10**(26): p. 21861–21875.

288. Wiemann, M., et al., Silver nanoparticles in the lung: Toxic effects and focal accumulation of silver in remote organs. *Nanomaterials*, 2017. **7**(12): p. 441.

289. Tang, J., et al., Influence of silver nanoparticles on neurons and blood-brain barrier via subcutaneous injection in rats. *Applied Surface Science*, 2008. **255**(2): p. 502–504.

290. Steinmetz, N.F., Viral nanoparticles as platforms for next-generation therapeutics and imaging devices. *Nanomedicine: Nanotechnology, Biology and Medicine*, 2010. **6**(5): p. 634–641.

291. Acharya, S. and S.K. Sahoo, PLGA nanoparticles containing various anticancer agents and tumour delivery by EPR effect. *Advanced Drug Delivery Reviews*, 2011. **63**(3): p. 170–183.

6

Nanobiosensors and Their Applications in Medical Diagnosis and Imaging

Naumih M. Noah and Peter M. Ndangili

Introduction

Early disease diagnosis and the monitoring of physical conditions are central to superior-quality health management since they are vital in providing better healthcare to minimize mortality rates as well as medical care costs (1). Making well-timed resolutions centred on swift diagnostics, smart data analysis, and informatics exploration can lead to better-quality standards of healthcare management (1). Medical diagnosis has significantly been enhanced due to the expansion of innovative techniques with the capability of performing very sensitive detection and quantifying various parameters (2). The analytical devices known as biosensors are capable of converting biological interaction into a measurable signal. They are therefore very important in medical diagnosis since they can directly determine the bioanalytical performance of an essay (1,3). The biosensors are also defined based on their biological or bioinspired receptor unit towards consistent analytes such as the deoxyribonucleic acid (DNA) of bacteria or viruses as well as proteins from antibodies or antigens of disease-ridden organisms (4).

Enhancing the performance of biosensors is very important to supporting human health and extending the human life span since numerous life-threatening diseases such as cancer, HIV, and viral diseases ought to be detected early to ensure their effective treatment (5). Also, the growing mandate for sensing an all-inclusive range of molecules at low detection limits and with high selectivity has inspired the expansion of a class of devices incorporating nanoscale materials, biological elements, and innovative materials, collectively called nanobiosensors (6). The use of nanotechnology in biosensors is an important development since the nanomaterials enhance and amplify the biosensor's signal which can reduce the diagnosis time as well as increase the accuracy and sensitivity of the biosensors (7,8).

DOI: 10.1201/9781003112068-6

Nanobiosensors are defined as portable and sensitive devices used to detect chemical and biological agents since they commonly consist of a nanomaterial that aids the bioreceptor immobilized onto the surface of a transducer (9,10). In nanobiosensors, nanostructures or nanomaterials are usually integrated into the biosensor by attachment to an appropriately modified platform (6). They, therefore, integrate the biological function and nanofabrication techniques and hence are useful for point-of-care diagnostics (10) since the nanomaterials increase the biosensor's effectiveness and sensitivity, due to their outstanding conductivity, surprising photoelectrochemical properties, and the prospect of miniaturizing the sensing platform (11). Different methods have been used to categorize nanobiosensors. These include categorization based on (10) samples such as blood, urine, and saliva, (9) biological elements such as antigens, antibodies, enzymes, or aptamers, (9) transducing techniques such as optical, colorimetric, electrochemical, mechanical, or magnetic, and (12) signal magnification processing methods (10). Figure 6.1 shows a schematic diagram of nanomaterial-based biosensors.

Various Nanobiosensors and Their Application in Medical Diagnosis and Imaging

Nanobiosensors as defined above are essentially sensors made up of nanomaterials. The small size of the nanomaterials brings most of their fundamental atoms at or near the surface enabling them to play a vital and effective role in the biosensor sensing mechanism (13). The efficient signal capture of the biological recognition event in biosensors has affected biosensor development in terms of sensitivity and selectivity (4). To improve the efficiency of the biosensors and to lower their detection limits, nanomaterials have been used, due to their capability of improving the immobilization of the bioreceptor at faster rates and their ability to act as transduction elements (4). Integrating the nanomaterials devices with electrical systems has given rise to nanoelectromechanical systems with enhanced sensitivity and low detection limits (13) for advanced diagnostics and daily routine tests (2). Various nanomaterials have been explored to improve the biological signalling and transduction mechanisms of biosensors based on their electronic and mechanical properties (13). The next section explores the use of nanoparticles, nanotubes, nanowires, and quantum dots in biosensors and their applications in medical diagnosis and imaging.

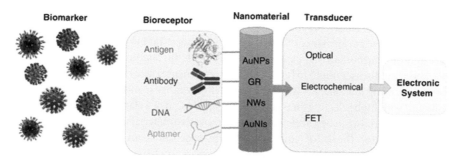

Figure 6.1 A schematic diagram representing a nanobiosensor with all its components. Adapted from (11), an open-access article.

Nanoparticle-Based Biosensors in Medical Diagnosis and Imaging

Nanoparticles have distinctive and size-dependent properties which can be controlled, meaning the nanoparticles have various applications in medicine and pharmacology (14). For example, they are associated with the design of specific nanostructures suitable for use as novel diagnostic devices and as therapeutic modalities (14) as well as use in scattering imaging techniques bringing valuable enhancements to standard imaging techniques (15). Metal nanoparticles from noble metals such as gold, silver, and platinum, although they are chemically inert in their macroscale form, exhibit exceptional physiochemical features at the nanoscale (16) and hence have very numerous beneficial properties that make them useful in transducers for biosensors (6). They have been extensively used as supportive electrode materials leading to an evolution of electron transfer rates and surface-to-volume ratio, thus permitting the immobilization of abundant amounts of the bio-receptors, moderating the non-specific binding (NSB) of proteins, with a consequent enhancement of the analytical response of the device (11). This section of the book chapter focuses on the application of some of these metal nanoparticles in biosensors for medical diagnosis and imaging.

Silver Nanoparticle-Based Biosensors for Medical Diagnosis and Imaging

Silver nanoparticles (AgNPs) have various valued optical properties for novel tactics in sensing and imaging applications, presenting an extensive variety of detection modes including colorimetric, scattering, and surface-enhanced Raman spectroscopy (SERS) techniques among others, at exceptionally low detection limits (15). They have tunable and exceptional plasmonic properties and exhibit high thermal and electrical conductivities with sharper extinction bands (5). Due to these features, they have been actively used in medical diagnosis and imaging, drug delivery, and as antimicrobial agents (5). In biosensing, for example, probe-conjugated AgNPs have shown highly efficient detection of clinical biomarkers for disease diagnosis (5).

The localized surface plasmon resonance (LSPR) characteristic of many metal nanoparticles such as AgNPs is normally produced when the incident photon frequency reverberates with the combined oscillation of unrestricted electrons (17,18) leading to an LSPR extinction spectrum, that can be monitored in the ultraviolet (UV)–visible region. This spectrum depends on the structure, size, shape, positioning, and local dielectric environment of the nanoparticles (17). For example, the peak wavelength of the LSPR extinction spectrum (λmax) is extremely sensitive to even small variations in the local refractive index close to the surface of the nanoparticle prompted by biomolecular interactions (19) enabling the nanoparticles to serve in biosensors. For example, a study by Zhao and co-workers reports a reusable AgNPs-based LSPR biosensor for the quantitative detection of serum squamous cell carcinoma (SCCa) antigen in cervical cancer patients (18). Using nanosphere lithography technology, the authors fabricated the AgNPs-based LSPR biosensor chip and functionalized it via several steps for selective and specific detection of biomolecular interaction as illustrated in Figure 6.2a. They then incubated the nanobiosensors in diverse standard concentrations of SCCa solution which ranged from 0.1 pM to 10,000 pM under optimum conditions and recorded the peak shifts of the obtained LSPR extinction spectra. Their results as shown in Figure 6.2b indicated a stepwise increase in the LSPR maximum wavelength ($\Delta\lambda$max) values with increasing SCCa concentrations with the linear logarithm

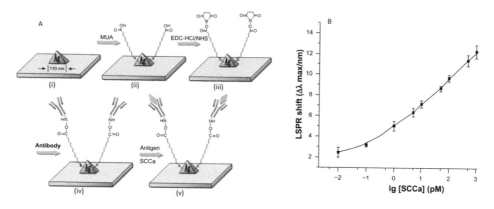

Figure 6.2 A schematic diagram showing an AgNPs-based biosensor for the detection of SCCa (a) and (b) the calibration curve of LSPR shift versus the logarithm of SCCa concentration. Reproduced from (18), an open-access article.

of concentrations within 0.1 pM to 1,000 pM which was better than that of commercial ELISA kits (1.75 pM to 115pM) (18).

Gold Nanoparticle-Based Biosensors for Medical Diagnosis and Imaging

Gold nanoparticles (AuNPs) are commonly used in medical biosensing applications owing to their remarkable optical/electrical properties, exceptional biocompatibility, catalytic properties, and comparatively easy synthetic pathways (11,20,21). They normally play different roles in the biosensing process depending on the transduction mode of the biosensor such as optical and electrochemical nanobiosensors (11). For the optical sensing modalities, the surface plasmon resonance (SPR) has attracted the most intensive research since the AuNPs are considered capable of amplifying the SPR signal (22) which is normally established on the molecular interaction of a receptor and a target analyte (23). This fact was proven by Makaraviciute et al. whose study showed a 3.5 times amplification of the analytical signal by considering protein G for site-directed antibody immobilization as compared to randomly oriented antibodies (24). AuNPs have been used to amplify an SPR signal for a biosensor developed for the fast and sensitive detection of cardiac troponin T (cTnT) in serum samples as reported by Pawula et al. (25). The authors used both direct and sandwich immunoassay formats where they conjugated the AuNPs to the anti-cTnT detection antibody. Their results indicated an enhancement of the SPR immunosensor signal which showed good reproducibility for the cTnT detection in the concentration range of 25–1,000 ng/mL and 5–400 ng/mL for the direct and sandwich immunoassays respectively (25) suggesting that the SPR immunosensor could be used for the early diagnosis of myocardial infarction (MI).

The localized surface plasmon resonance (LSPR) mechanism where the bio/chemical interface on the surface of metallic nanoparticles leads to an enhancement of the refractive index of local medium occasioning a shift of the resonant wavelength has been exploited in the development of biosensors for the recognition of protein biomarkers (26–28). A study by Lee et al. reported a nanoplasmonic biosensor based on a single AuNP and antibody-antigen binding activity for the detection of cancer biomarkers such as α-fetoprotein

(AFP), carcinoembryonic antigen (CEA), and prostate-specific antigen (PSA) (29). Their nanobiosensor exhibited exceptional selectivity and sensitivity with a detection limit of 91 fM, 94 fM, and 10 fM for AFP, CEA, and PSA from patient-mimicked serum, respectively (29).

AuNPs are also said to provide exceptional platforms for the improvement of colorimetric biosensors since they can be easily functionalized, displaying diverse colours subject to their size, shape, and state of aggregation (30). As such, they have been reported to have been used in the development of a colorimetric nanobiosensor for the clinical detection of prostate-specific antigen (PSA) based on ascorbic acid (AA)-induced *in situ* formations of AuNPs and Cu^{2+}-catalyzed oxidation of AA (31). Similarly, a study by Shayesteh et al. reported an innovative label-free colorimetric AuNPs-based aptasensor for the sensitive detection of PSA tumour marker in human serum adsorbed non-thiolated poly-adenine aptamer (polyA Apt) (32). The fabricated AuNPs-based aptasensor indicated a linear detection range of 0.1–100 ng/ml with a limit of detection of 20 pg/mL indicating that the aptasensor could be applied to real samples for the fast screening of PSA (32).

Due to their higher surface area as compared to flat surfaces, the AuNPs can be used as novel immobilization electrochemical transducers as well as for signal amplification (33). A study by Brondani et al. (34) reported a label-free electrochemical immunosensor based on ((E)-4-[(4-decyloxyphenyl)diazenyl]-1-methyl pyridinium iodide), an ionic organic molecule as a redox probe, and chitosan-stabilized gold nanoparticles (CTS-AuNPs) as a green platform for the immobilization of monoclonal anti-cTnT antibody for the detection of cTnT. The authors used cyclic and square wave voltammetry to detect the presence of cTnT antigens following their interaction with the anti-cTnT antibody which was immobilized on the surface of the immunosensor (34). Their results indicated that interaction resulted in a decrease in the electrochemical analytical signal which was proportional to the concentration of cTnT antigens present at a linearity range of 0.20 to 1.00 ng/mL cTnT, with a calculated limit of detection of 0.10 ng/ mL which was better when compared to other immunosensors reported in the literature (34).

A study by Rahi et al. reports an electrochemical label-free aptasensor for the detection of the prostate-specific antigen (PSA) (35). In their work, they electrodeposited gold nanorods with the help of arginine as a soft template and used them as a transducer for the immobilization of an aptamer of the PSA. Their AuNPs-based aptasensor indicated a linear detection range of 0.125–200 ng/mL and 50 pg/mL as the limit of detection which was successfully used to detect PSA in blood serum samples of healthy persons and patients (35).

The AuNPs can also be conjugated with other nanomaterials such as carbon nanotubes (CNTs) to further improve their binding capacity and hence their biosensing capability (36). For example, nanohybrids of AuNPs and CNTs, as well as gold nanoislands, have been synthesized and found to offer a more effective immobilization matrix for numerous biosensing applications such as growth hormone detection (36). Likewise, a study by Heydari-Bafrooei and co-workers reported ultrasensitive label-free electrochemical aptasensors for the detection of PSA in serum based on reduced graphene (rGO) multiwalled CNT (rGO-MWCNT)/AuNPs nanocomposite modified electrode (37). This modified electrode was found to be the most sensitive aptasensing platform for the determination of PSA with an exceptionally low detection limit of 1.0pg/mL PSA and within the linear detection range of 0.005–20 ngmL^{-1} and 0.005–100 ngmL^{-1} for differential pulse voltammetry (DPV) and electrochemical impedance spectroscopy (EIS) calibration curves, respectively, as

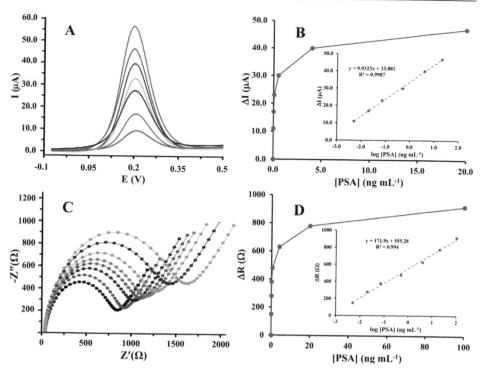

Figure 6.3 (A) Differential pulse voltammetry (DPV) curves and (C) Nyquist plots of aptamer-immobilized rGOMWCNT/AuNPs for PSA detection at different concentrations. Linear calibration curve for (B) ΔI and (D) ΔR vs. log (CPSA/ng mL⁻¹), where CPSA is the PSA concentration. Reproduced with permission from (37).

illustrated in Figure 6.3 (37). The nanosensor was also found to exhibit an exceptional anti-interference capability concerning co-existing molecules with decent stability, sensitivity, and reproducibility (37).

AuNPs in combination with silver nanoparticles (AgNPs) have been utilized in the fabrication of a surface-enhanced Raman spectroscopy (SERS) biosensor for the detection of micro ribonucleic acid (miRNA) with a detection limit of 3 fM as reported by Shao et al. (38).

AuNPs have also been utilized in the development of a nano-polymer chain reaction (PCR) biosensor for the diagnosis of foot and mouth disease virus (FMDV) using thiol-linked oligonucleotides that recognize the conserved 3D gene of FMDV, as reported by Hamdy et al. (39). Their nanobiosensors indicated 94.5% efficiency and 100% specificity as shown in Figure 6.4, and hence they can be suitable for use in quarantine stations and farms for the rapid diagnosis of FMDV in endemic areas (39).

Gold nanoparticles and nanostructures have also been used in the sensing of drugs such as epirubicin, an anticancer chemotherapy drug (40), and neurotransmitters such as dopamine (41). Owing to their stress-free fabrication, chemical solidity, exceptional biocompatibility, and flexible optical properties, AuNPs have also been used in bioimaging to provide high-resolution images which do not necessitate the usage of radioactive contrast agents (42). Larger AuNPs have been reported to demonstrate sturdier scattering effectiveness than smaller AuNPs (42,43), and in contrast to fluorophores, the light-scattering AuNPs are not photo-bleachable making them very reliable contrast agents for bioimaging (42). Based

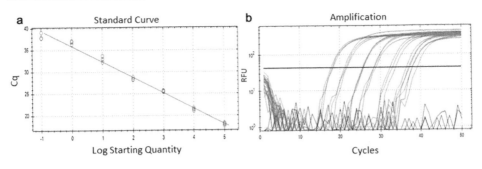

Figure 6.4 The standard curve (a) and amplification plot (b) of the rRT-PCR assay using AuNPs-FMDV biosensor (400 nM primer) with serial dilution RNA standard of FMDV 3D gene show Eff. % = 94.5% and R2 = 0.989 and slope = −3.544. Reproduced with slight modification from (39), an open-access article.

on the two main imaging modalities which detect the backscattering of AuNPs: dark field confocal imaging (DFCI) and optical coherence tomography (OCT), various AuNPs have been instigated as DF optical contrast proxies for cancer cell imaging by functionalizing their surface with ligand binding to cell surface receptors (44). For example, Wan and co-workers reported a real-time light scattering tracking of AuNPs-bioconjugated respiratory syncytial virus to visualize its infection of HEp-2 cells (45).

Graphene-Based Biosensors for Medical Diagnosis and Imaging

Graphene is a two-dimensional (2D) nanomaterial, that plays a central role in the field of biosensors due to its extraordinary physical, optical, and electrochemical properties (46–49). Different kinds of graphene exist including pristine graphene and functionalized graphene such as graphene oxide (GO), reduced graphene oxide (rGO), and graphene-based quantum dots (GQDs) (50–52). The graphene-based biosensors can be developed by assembling functioned graphene materials such as GO, rGO, and GQDs onto the biosensor surface for better assembling of molecular receptors which improves the performance of the biosensor by increasing the surface area and the distinctive π–π orbital interaction on the interface (53). The graphene-based biosensors have also been developed by using the graphene materials as excellent carriers for the construction of novel nanocomposites which leads to the amplification of the biosensor signal (54,55). Electrochemical and electrochemiluminescent biosensors with the improved capability of combining with different biomolecules with higher surface area and excellent biocompatibility have been constructed using graphene nanomaterials and antibodies (54,56,57). This has been done by utilizing the strong cross-linking between the carboxylic acid groups on graphene materials and the amine groups of the antibodies to assemble the antibody on the biosensor interface (58,59).

A study by Mao and co-workers reports an amperometric immunosensor for the detection of prostate-specific antigen (PSA) using a nanocomposite film of graphene sheets-methylene blue-chitosan as an electrode material (60). The nanocomposite was found to show high binding affinity to the electrode and was used to immobilize the PSA antibody which was monitored using cyclic voltammetry (CV). The results showed a decrease of the peak current with the PSA concentration which was induced by the specific antigen-antibody interaction at a linear range of between 0.05 and 5.00 ng/mL and with a limit

151

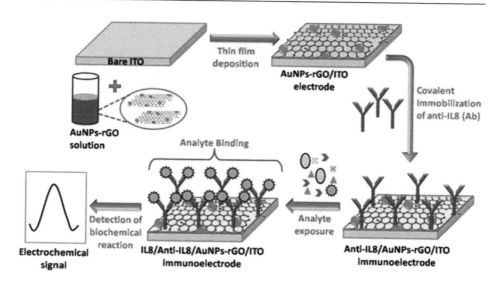

Figure 6.5 A schematic diagram representing the fabrication of Au NPs-rGO-based immunosensor. Adapted with permission from (62).

of detection of 13 pg/mL (60). Similarly, another study by Wu and co-workers reports a label-free electrochemiluminescent (ECL) immunosensor for the detection of PSA based on aminated graphene quantum dots and carboxyl graphene quantum dots (61). They modified the electrode surface with Au/Ag-rGO for the adsorption of the PSA antibody and then combined a large amount of the amminated GQDs and the carboxyl GQDs on the electrode surface for the ECL signal amplification. The ECL intensity was found to decrease linearly with the logarithm of PSA concentration in the range of 1 pg/mL~10 ng/mL with a limit of detection of 0.29 pg/mL (61).

Another study that utilized highly stable gold nanoparticles-reduced graphene oxide (AuNPs-rGO) composite as the transducer matrix has been reported for the noninvasive detection of interleukin-8 (IL8), an oral cancer biomarker, as illustrated in Figure 6.5 (62). The study demonstrated that the synergy between the rGO and the AuNPs led to an improved electron transfer which allowed the immunosensor to exhibit a rapid response and high sensitivity with a good experimental linear dynamic range as well as reusability and stability of up to three months (62).

Graphene nanomaterials such as graphene quantum dots (GQD) and nanographene have been used in medical bioimaging both *in vivo* and *in vitro* because of their exceptional optical properties including near-infrared photoluminescence, magnetic resonance, and characteristic Raman bands among others (8). A study by Liu et al. reported the ability of propidium iodide (PI)-GO to enter into the nuclei and stain the DNA/RNA of living human breast cancer cells MCF-7 (63). In their study, they found that the PI alone could not penetrate the cellular membrane, indicating that the GO enabled the PI delivery for the live cell staining (63).

Carbon Nanotube-Based Biosensors for Medical Diagnosis and Imaging

Carbon nanotubes (CNTs) are a carbon allotrope that are either single or rolled-up graphene sheets (64). Based on the number of the graphene sheets, CNTs can be grouped as either single-walled carbon nanotubes (SWCNTs), with only a single graphene sheet wrapped, or multiwalled carbon nanotubes (MWCNTs), with more than one sheet, wrapped concentrically (64). CNTs have been synthesized mostly using the chemical vapour deposition (CVD) technique as described in the literature (65,66).

CNTs have unique mechanical, electrochemical, and thermal properties which have made them gain intensive attention. Their surface can be functionalized with various bio/chemical species paving the way for their application in medical diagnosis and imaging since this not only overcomes their hydrophobicity that tends to form very lethal aggregates (67) but also contributes to the variation of the biocompatibility of the CNTs themselves (67). The hollow interior of the CNTs as well as their excellent physical properties and their enhanced permeability and retention (EPR) capability make them appropriate for use in cancer diagnosis since they can penetrate tumour tissues (68). Also due to the non-covalent $\pi-\pi$ stacking of CNTs, they can be used to load hydrophobic drugs ensuring directed drug delivery that is assured by the outer surface functionalization which is crucial to avoid healthy tissue damage (64). The extraordinary sensitivity of CNTs guarantees that they can serve as a perfect material for highly sensitive nanobiosensor devices as reported by Thirumalral and co-workers (69). In their study, they developed an electrochemical biosensor based on the poly-l-lysine (PLL) electro-polymerized on the surface of functionalized MWCNT for the detection of palmatine content in human serum and urine samples at a linear response range of 0.5 µM to 425 µM and a detection limit (LOD) of 0.12 µM (69). Another study reports the detection of Tau protein using antibody functionalized MWCNTs with a significantly enhanced response which is normally challenging to obtain especially with the protein alone while using the conventional unconjugated sandwich assays (70).

Another study by Rezaei et al. (71) reported the use of carboxylated MWCNTs-whiskered nanofibres in the development of an electrochemical immunosensor for cardiac troponin (cTn1) with a wide detection range for cTn1 of between 0.5 and 20 ng/mL and with a detection limit of 0.04 ng/mL. This detection range showed the clinical borderline for a normal person to the concentration present in myocardial infarction patients indicating its potential for point-of-care testing (71).

In addition to application in medical diagnosis, engineered CNTs have also been reported to act as exceptional adjuvant contrast agents (CA) for various imaging techniques (72).

Nanowire-Based Biosensors

Nanowire-based biosensors comprise nanowires or nanofibres at a nanoscopic scale, incorporated into sensing devices. They are considered the most powerful nanomaterials in medical applications, owing to their ability to allow for electrical label-free detection of species (73) and fast detection as well as high data delivery (74). Their synthesis from semiconductors and control of dopant type can easily be achieved (75). Furthermore, the modification of surfaces of nanowires has been shown to increase their sensitivity to biological species (76). The bioimaging principle of nanowires involves the transduction of molecular interaction through a wire into an ion-sensitive field-effect transistor (FET) or a memristor electrochemical signal (74). The detection of FET sensors is in the range of 10^{-15} M (fM) to 10^{-9} M (nM) (77), while that of the memristor is in the range of 10^{-18} M (aM) to 10^{-15} (fM) (78). The FET bioimaging devices comprise three electrodes: (a) source (S), (b) drain (D), and (c) gate (G); while memristor devices are two-electrode systems, comprising S and D only (79). The source and the drain act as a bridge to the nanowire channel, while the gate serves as the reference electrode for modulation of the electronic properties of the nanowire material. Suitable nanowires such as those of silicon can be doped positively or negatively to obtain p-type or n-type nanowires, respectively (80). The interaction between nanowire-immobilized and soluble biomolecules results in the transfer of quantifiable charges into the wire in the form of change on the conductance (for FET) or change in voltage gap (for memristor) (74).

Fabrication of Nanowire Sensors

Effective biosensing using nanowires is achieved through the assembly of nanowire arrays, most of which are vertical nanowire arrays (81). These vertical nanowire arrays are vertically and uniformly distributed arrays and may have solid, hollow, or hybrid structures. They are made of materials such as silicon and silicon dioxide as well as metal oxides which include Al_2O_3, TiO_2, ZnO_2, and IrO_2 (82). Others are carbon, platinum, and gold nanowire arrays (81). Nanowire sensors are fabricated using two main approaches: (a) bottom-up, and (b) top-down methods (83). The bottom-up method is preferred because it produces high-quality nanowires. The method starts with the packing of atoms and molecules along the energy priority direction. The materials are then assembled into nanowires from smaller units, followed by catalytic growth of nanowires using the chemical vapour deposition method, via the vapour-liquid-solid mechanism (84), atomic layer deposition (85), or metal-organic vapour phase epitaxy (86). The synthesized nanowires are suspended in ethanol and deposited into a silicon substrate. This is followed by spin-coating a photoresist into the substrate, after which the metal electrodes are patterned by the lift-off method. The last step involves passivation and surface modification to introduce bioconjugation groups. This method allows for variation of the cross-sectional shape, giving round, square, and triangular-shaped nanowires (87). However, the method is associated with a random orientation of nanowires, which gives rise to poor uniformity and consequently low-rate nanowire sensors. This calls for additional synthesis steps to improve their orientation. These steps include contact printing (88), microfluidic flow (89), Langmuir-Blodgett (90), blown bubble (91), and electric field (92), among others.

On the other hand, top-down synthetic routes are achieved by the use of block materials via advanced engraving and etching processes (93). This mainly involves non-optical electron beam (94), ion beam (95), X-ray (96) interference, or holography lithography techniques, metal-assisted chemical etching (93), and reactive ion etching (97) The patterns of the nanowires are obtained through a series of masking steps. This method results in nanowires with higher mechanical reliability compared to the bottom-up method (81).

Characterization

The surface morphology, size, size distribution, and orientations of the synthesized nanowires are elucidated using atomic force microscopy (98), X-ray diffraction spectroscopy, scanning electron microscopy, and transmission electron microscopic techniques (81). The scanning electron microscopy and transmission electron microscopy equipment are sometimes coupled with energy dispersive X-ray analysers for the determination of the elemental composition of the synthesized materials (81). Fourier transform infrared spectroscopy is used to study the bioconjugation between the nanowires and the biomolecules (99).

Depending on the method of detection to be used, further characterization methods are applied. For instance, if the method to be used is electrochemical, electrochemical techniques such as cyclic voltammetry and electrochemical impedance spectroscopy (100) are used to determine electron transfer and resistance processes. X-ray photoelectron spectroscopy may also be used to characterize the sensor platform. For optical detection methods, ultraviolet-visible and fluorescence spectroscopic techniques are used (101,102).

Specific Applications in Bioimaging

Nanowire sensors have been developed for the rapid detection of DNA. For instance, Zhang et al. demonstrated successful near-infrared photoluminescence detection of thrombin and DNA using gold nanorods over gallium arsenide nanohorn arrays (103). Silicon-based nanowires functionalized with antigen-specific antibodies have been used as biomarkers for cancer diagnosis. Reports of Tzouvadaki and co-workers (78) demonstrated the successful detection of prostate-specific antigen using DNA aptamers on silicon nanowires on a memristive sensor. These authors attained a detection limit of 23 aM. A highly selective and stable DNA sensor was developed by Zhang and co-workers using ZnO nanowires on graphite microfibre electrodes (100). The authors achieved a dynamic detection range between 10^{-2} pM and 10^{-1} µM and an ultralow detection limit of 3.3×10^{-3} pM. A nanowire-mediated lysis of cells for microbial cell identification was demonstrated by Yasui and co-workers (104).

Significant applications of nanowire sensors have been extended to the capture of circulating tumour cells, cellular electrical signals, and mechanotransduction sensing (81). The interaction between cell surfaces and nanowire array structures is associated with high cell capture affinity, thereby facilitating the distinction of normal and abnormal cells in whole blood samples (105,106). Zhang et al. developed indium-titanium oxide hierarchical nanowire arrays for efficient cancer cell capture (107). The capture of breast cancer cells was demonstrated by Liu and co-workers using polystyrene nanotube substrate (108). Others include antibody free isolation of tumour cells using a TiO_2/ZnO branched microtube array (109), and intracellular regulation and monitoring of circulating tumour cells using a multifunctional branched nanostraw-electroporation platform (110).

Although significant achievements have been made in nanowire sensors for bioimaging, there are limitations in the clinical detection of cancer. These limitations include the need for individual sensor calibration, the presence of salts that decrease the Debye length, and lack of multiplex sensing capabilities since nanowires are limited to three analytes only (74).

Quantum Dot-Based Biosensors

Quantum dots are inorganic semiconducting materials, composed of between 9 and 51 atoms and whose diameter is between 3 and 9 nm (111). They are mainly composed of core materials of different metal-non-metal combinations such as groups II-IV, IV-VI, or III-V (112). Medical imaging applications of quantum dots from these groups are met with challenges of insolubility, bio-incompatibility, and toxicity. Group II–IV quantum dots such as CdTe and CdSe are particularly toxic due to the release of Cd^{2+} from the material as a result of photolysis and oxidation. The toxicity of cadmium-based quantum dots is influenced by their size, charge, and coating ligands, as well as oxidative, photolytic, and mechanical stability (112). Other toxic quantum dots are those of lead and arsenic. Another challenge of the quantum dots is their rapid elimination from the body system through the reticuloendothelial system (RES) or via entrapment by the liver and spleen (113). This results in poor imaging quality and enhanced background noise (112). These challenges have been addressed by changing their composition, as well as introducing surface functionalities on the quantum dots surface. These modifications are usually designed carefully so that the desired properties of the quantum dots are not compromised. For instance, the conjugation of silicon quantum dots with polymers has been shown to lower their potential toxicity in biological applications. Moreover, when quantum dots are suitably functionalized, they exhibit high stability compared to organic molecules (114,115). To ensure long retention periods in the body, the quantum dots are masked to make them undetectable by the reticuloendothelial system. This is achieved through the introduction of protecting and targeting ligands such as lipoproteins and peptides. They can also be prepared in an aqueous form to adapt to the bio-environment (112).

Owing to the presence of tens of thousands of delocalized chemically bonded individual atoms in a single quantum dot, their tolerance against photon-induced damage is greatly enhanced (116). The use of quantum dots as signal reporters in medical imaging started with the report of Orte et al., who demonstrated the use of functionalized quantum dots for the detection of intracellular pH changes, in conjunction with fluorescence lifetime imaging (117). The signal in this report was the quantum dot's photoluminescence decay time, and improved sensitivity was recorded compared to fluorescence pH dyes. Since then, other quantum dot-based imaging applications have been developed for intracellular Ca^{2+} (118) and K^+ (119), among others. The imaging of intracellular Ca^{2+} is permeated by Forster resonance energy transfer (FRET) between the donor quantum dots and red-emitting $CaRuByCa^{2+}$ dye receptor, attached to the surface of the quantum dot (118). If this nano-assembly is further functionalized with cell-penetrating proteins, cytosolic delivery properties are conferred. Consequently, this can allow for the resolution of cross-membrane Ca^{2+} transients in baby hamster kidney cells (BHK cells), an advancement that opens new possibilities for exploring microdomain Ca^{2+} signalling events. Recent studies have explored the application of quantum dots as radiosensitizers and near-infrared optical *in vivo* and *in vitro* imaging devices for the viewing and treatment of tumour immune responses (120), malignant detectors (121), tumour-specific receptors, and sentinel lymph nodes (122,123).

Silicon quantum dots have received extensive applications in bioimaging. This is because they are characterized by resistance to photobleaching, high quantum yields, and a wide emission range from visible to infrared regions (112). Their sizes can easily be modulated to below 10 nm. They have found wide applications as fluorescence probes for medical imaging due to their non-toxicity, and enviro-friendly nature (124). Silicon quantum dots degrade into silicic acid when used for *in vivo* applications (125). The silicic acid is excreted through the urine. On the other hand, silicon quantum dots are considered many times safer than cadmium-based quantum dots in *in vitro* applications (126). Despite their attractive features in bioimaging applications, silicon quantum dots are not biocompatible, have unstable photoluminescence, and are insoluble in aqueous media. This results from their synthesis of solvents such as octane and styrene, which are hydrophobic. These challenges have to be addressed for successful bioimaging applications. Reports of Tilley and Yamamoto (127) demonstrated that the surface modification of silicon quantum dots with poly (acrylic acid) and allylamine results in water-soluble quantum dots whose fixed cell labelling is successful.

Synthesis of Quantum Dots

Several methods have been reported for the synthesis of quantum dots. These include hydrothermal/microwave-assisted methods, organometallic methods, and synthesis from aqueous solutions. Each of these methods is briefly discussed below.

Hydrothermal Methods

This method involves loading the reaction reagents into a hermetic container, which is heated to super-critical temperatures (128). The high temperature ensures the separation of nucleation processes from crystal formation, leading to reduced surface defects and short reaction time (99). Besides the reduced surface defects, the quantum dots produced by this method have a narrow size distribution.

Microwave-Assisted Methods

This method is similar to the hydrothermal method in the sense that the synthesis is temperature-driven. Whereas heated hermetic containers are used in hydrothermal methods, microwave-assisted methods use microwave irradiation as their heat source. Water is usually used as a solvent in this method, which is irradiated to temperatures above 100°C, yielding homogeneous quantum dots, with good quantum yield. This is the most common method reported for the synthesis of carbon dots (129–132).

Organometallic Synthesis Methods

This method produces quantum dots through the pyrolysis of organometallic reagents following their injection into hot coordinating solvents at temperatures ranging between 250°C and 300°C (133). Ligands such as tri-n-octyl phosphine oxide (TOPO) are used to control the quantum dot growth and annealing of the core materials in the coordinating solvents (134). The method leads to the formation of monodispersed quantum dots with different sizes and high quantum yields. The modulation of these properties is achieved through varying the synthesis temperature and time. This is an established synthesis method and is widely used. Some quantum dots synthesized by this method are those of cadmium telluride (134), cadmium selenide using dimethyl cadmium, and Bis (trimethylsilyl) selenium as the organometallic precursors (112).

Aqueous Synthetic Methods

The synthesis of quantum dots in aqueous solutions started with the work of Rajh and co-workers (135) who demonstrated the successful synthesis of thiol-capped CdTe quantum dots in an aqueous solution. Since then, many quantum dot architectures have been synthesized using various precursors. The precursors may be commercial compounds such as ionic cadmium perchlorate and aluminium tellurite, for the synthesis of CdTe quantum dots. They may also be prepared separately, followed by their introduction into reaction chambers for nucleation. This method has been used for the synthesis of ZnSe (136), PdTe (137), Ga_2Se_3 (138), Ga_2Te_3, and binary quantum dots, as well as ternary quantum dot systems such as zinc-gallium-selenide (139) and zinc-gallium telluride. The synthesis is usually performed in the presence of stabilizing ligands such as mercaptopropionic acid (140), glutathione, or hydrothiol-containing surfactants. This is a low-cost method, can be performed at laboratory temperatures, and is environmentally friendly. The use of mercaptopropionic acid, glutathione, or hydrothiol-containing surfactant capping agents results in soluble and biocompatible quantum dots, without further surface modifications. The disadvantage of this method is that thiol-capped quantum dots have a wide size distribution and poor stability in aqueous solutions, have low quantum yields, and have broad full width at half maxima.

To suit bioimaging applications, post-synthesis procedures are carried out to ensure stability, solubility, and biocompatibility, among others. This procedure is not often required if aqueous synthesis methods are used. Studies have shown that some quantum dots, especially those that contain cadmium, pose cytotoxic effects to the human body. The surface coating of these quantum dots has been shown to significantly reduce their cytotoxicity. To address this, core-shell synthetic procedures are used, where the quantum dots are coated with an inorganic layer of another quantum dot, whose composition is safe and whose band gap is wider than that of the core material. The introduction of this extra layer calls for further surface modification so that other properties such as solubility and biocompatibility are conferred.

To use quantum dots in biological systems, they have to be soluble in aqueous solvents. This property may be conferred directly if the quantum dots are synthesized in aqueous media. Alternatively, the quantum dots are synthesized in organic media, followed by ligand exchange procedures that lead to the introduction of hydrophilic groups on the quantum dot surface. The introduction of hydrophilic groups is advantageous in that it also confers biocompatibility properties on the quantum dots. The characterization techniques for quantum dots are similar to those of nanowires discussed above.

Specific Applications in Bioimaging

In Vivo *Imaging*

The *in vivo* imaging of isolated circulating tumour cells and stem cell tracking are important procedures in cancer diagnosis and immune system monitoring (101). The imaging of individual cell migration was demonstrated by Bouccara and co-workers using Zn–Cu–In–Se/ZnS core/shell quantum dots (102). These quantum dots exhibited long-time fluorescence (150 ns) in the near-infrared region. Coupled with a time-gated detection, the authors achieved discrimination between signal and short-time fluorescence. The time-gated fluorescence imaging technique allows a delay between pulsed excitation and fluorescence emission detection, whose photons are detected from the longer lifetime probes, while at the same time rejecting those from short lifetime fluorophores (101). Time-gated Forster resonance energy transfer between terbium complexes and semiconductor quantum dots conjugated with antibodies of epidermal growth factor receptor allows sensitive imaging of intracellular and extracellular interactions (141). Biocompatible $(Zn)CuInS_2$ were used as non-toxic and superior probes for imaging human breast cancer cells using the time-gated fluorescence technique (142). The probes were found to suppress autofluorescence and improve the signal:noise ratio by orders of magnitude. For the detection of isolated tumour cells circulating in the bloodstream, Bouccara and co-workers developed and optimized the optical properties of ZnCuInSe/ZnS quantum dots (101). They coated the quantum dots with an imidazole zwitterionic multidentate block copolymer, to prolong the stability of the quantum dots in the live cell's cytoplasm. The quantum dots were labelled with erythrocytes and lymphoma cells and injected into the bloodstream. The authors were able to image and count the quantum dot-labelled cells in blood vessels at low velocities (mm s^{-1}).

Carbon quantum dots possess high chemical stability, have excellent fluorescence, and are easy to synthesize (98). They also exhibit high imaging resolution, long-term detection, low invasiveness, and unique biocompatibility (143,144). They have been established as safe non-toxic nanoprobes for efficient imaging of both *in vivo* and *in vitro* diagnosis. Apart from mouse fibroblast cells and human prostate cancer cells, carbon quantum dots have been found to efficiently label cells and zebrafish (98). They have been proposed as potential optical probes for human clinical trials.

Recent advances have witnessed the development of gelatin quantum dots for imaging a variety of bacterial cells (99). Successful imaging of *Escherichia coli* and *Staphylococcus aureus*, yeast cells including *Candida albicans*, *C. krusei*, *C. parapsilosis*, and *C. tropicalis*, mycelial fungi including *Aspergillus flavus* and *A. fumigatus* cells, and cancer cell lines A549, HEK293, and L929 by these authors presents the potential use of gelatin quantum dots in clinical diagnosis.

In Vitro *Imaging*

The application of quantum dots in bioimaging started after demonstrating that these nanomaterials can be used to label cells. Consequently, many applications have reported the use of quantum dots as cell labels. These include the use of capped CdSe/Zns quantum dots by Jaiswal and co-workers (145), who labelled HeLa cells. The authors successfully achieved uptake of the quantum dots by the endothelial cells and were able to realize selective labelling of the cell surface proteins with antibody-conjugated quantum dots. On their part, Li et al. synthesized 3-mercaptopropionic acid-capped CdS quantum dots and used them for imaging *Salmonella typhimurium* cells (146). Water-soluble quantum dots of PbS and PbSe have also been used for cell labelling (147). The authors achieved water solubility by the use of carboxylic groups as surface functionalizing materials. The quantum dots obtained exhibited emissions in the near-infrared region and permitted the labelling and imaging of colon cancer cells.

Advances have been made in bioimaging using quantum dots by the identification of specific biomolecules as biomarkers, which are then labelled using quantum dots for their continuous tracking. This allows for the progressive monitoring of cancer cells following the administration of drug therapies. Functionalized CdTe-coated silica quantum dots have been demonstrated as suitable biomarker labels for cell imaging (148). The authors used polyethylene glycol (PEG) grafted polyethyleneimine (PEI-g-PEG) to coat and solubilize the quantum dots via direct ligand exchange reactions. They established that the multivalent imine groups conferred solubility properties on the quantum dots. Further, the inclusion of the PEG in the capping surface prevented the penetration of Cd^{2+} into the living cells, thereby reducing cytotoxicity. It also improved the quantum dot's stability and biocompatibility. The quantum dots obtained penetrated cell membranes and were able to disrupt endosomal organelles in the living cells. The others observed that the synthesized quantum dots get integrated into the body through endocytosis and are stored in the vesicles. They then are released into the cytoplasm.

Conclusion and Future Perspective

Nanoparticles have emerged as a new class of materials for biomolecular and cellular imaging. Compared with organic dyes and bulk materials, nanoparticles possess unique optical and electronic properties, suitable for high-resolution imaging required in medical diagnosis. Their ability to allow for the modulation of their properties has opened possibilities for the assembly of a wide variety of technologies for biomedical diagnosis and imaging. For this reason, significant advances have been made in the development of nano-imaging technology. Specifically, metal nanoparticles, carbon nanotubes, graphene, nanowires, and quantum dots have been discussed in this chapter. These nanoparticles have great potential for applications in medical diagnosis and bioimaging.

However, there are limitations in the use of nanoparticles in *in vivo* imaging. The limitations arise from their cytotoxicity and hydrophobicity. Post-synthesis procedures have to be carried out to confer biocompatibility properties, ensure stability, reduce toxicity, and enhance target molecule binding capacity. Single-step synthesis procedures are therefore required to reduce the time and cost of synthesis. Another challenge of the use of nanoparticles in *in vivo* imaging, which needs to be addressed, is their clearance from the body. It was also noted that the success of one nano-assembly in the imaging of cells may not be generalized to all cells. This was exemplified by Tian and co-workers (98) whose carbon dots could tag all cells and zebrafish, but could not tag mouse fibroblast cells and human prostate cancer cells. Extensive research is therefore required for each type of cell to determine its success or lack of it.

References

1. Noah NM, Ndangili PM. Current trends of nanobiosensors for point-of-care diagnostics. *J Anal Methods Chem.* 2019;2019:2179718. Available from: https://doi.org/10.1155/2019/2179718

2. Chamorro-Garcia A, Merkoçi A. Nanobiosensors in diagnostics. *Nanobiomedicine.* 2016 Nov 24;3:1849543516663574–1849543516663574. Available from: https://pubmed.ncbi.nlm.nih.gov/29942385

3. Metkar SK, Girigoswami K. Diagnostic biosensors in medicine–A review. *Biocatal Agric Biotechnol.* 2019;17:271–83.

4. Holzinger M, Le Goff A, Cosnier S. Nanomaterials for biosensing applications: a review. *Frontiers in Chemistry.* 2014;2:63. Available from: https://www.frontiersin.org/article/10.3389/fchem.2014.00063

5. Tan P, Li H, Wang J, Gopinath SCB. Silver nanoparticle in biosensor and bioimaging: Clinical perspectives. *Biotechnol Appl Biochem.* 2020 Oct 11. Available from: https://doi.org/10.1002/bab.2045

6. Malekzad H, Zangabad PS, Mirshekari H, Karimi M, Hamblin MR. Noble metal nanoparticles in biosensors: Recent studies and applications. *Nanotechnol Rev.* 2017 Jun 27;6(3):301–29. Available from: https://pubmed.ncbi.nlm.nih.gov/29335674

7. Farshchi F, Hasanzadeh M. Nanomaterial based aptasensing of prostate specific antigen (PSA): Recent progress and challenges in efficient diagnosis of prostate cancer using biomedicine. *Biomed Pharmacother.* 2020 Dec;132:110878.

8. Gu H, Tang H, Xiong P, Zhou Z. Biomarkers-based biosensing and bioimaging with graphene for cancer diagnosis. *Nanomater (Basel, Switzerland).* 2019 Jan 21;9(1):130. Available from: https://pubmed.ncbi.nlm.nih.gov/30669634

9. Fox KE, Tran NL, Nguyen TA, Nguyen TT, Tran PA. Surface modification of medical devices at nanoscale—Recent development and translational perspectives. In: Yang L, Bhaduri SB, Webster TJBT-B in TM, eds. *Woodhead publishing series in biomaterials.* Academic Press; 2019. p. 163–89. Available from: https://www.sciencedirect.com/science/article/pii/B9780128134771000086

10. Vasile C. Chapter 1 - Polymeric nanomaterials: Recent developments, properties and medical applications. In: Vasile CBT-PN in N, ed. *Micro and nano technologies.* Elsevier; 2019. p. 1–66. Available from: https://www.sciencedirect.com/science/article/pii/B9780128139325000017

11. Antiochia R. Nanobiosensors as new diagnostic tools for SARS, MERS and COVID-19: From past to perspectives. *Microchim Acta.* 2020;187(12):639. Available from: https://doi.org/10.1007/s00604-020-04615-x

12. Luka G, Ahmadi A, Najjaran H, Alocilja E, DeRosa M, Wolthers K, et al. Microfluidics integrated biosensors: A leading technology towards lab-on-a-chip and sensing applications. *Sensors (Basel).* 2015 Dec;15(12):30011–31.

13. Malik P, Katyal V, Malik V, Asatkar A, Inwati G, Mukherjee TK. Nanobiosensors: Concepts and variations. *ISRN Nanomater.* 2013;2013:327435. Available from: https://doi.org/10.1155/2013/327435

14. Klębowski B, Depciuch J, Parlińska-Wojtan M, Baran J. Applications of noble metal-based nanoparticles in medicine. *Int J Mol Sci.* 2018 Dec 13;19(12):4031. Available from: https://pubmed.ncbi.nlm.nih.gov/30551592

15. Caro C. Silver nanoparticles: Sensing and imaging applications. In: Castillo PM, ed. *Silver nanoparticles.* Rijeka: IntechOpen; 2010. Available from: https://doi.org/10.5772/8513

16. Wu B, Kuang Y, Zhang X, Chen J. Noble metal nanoparticles/carbon nanotubes nanohybrids: Synthesis and applications. *Nano Today.* 2011;6(1):75–90.

17. Petryayeva E, Krull UJ. Localized surface plasmon resonance: Nanostructures, bioassays and biosensing--A review. *Anal Chim Acta.* 2011 Nov;706(1):8–24.

18. Zhao Q, Duan R, Yuan J, Quan Y, Yang H, Xi M. A reusable localized surface plasmon resonance biosensor for quantitative detection of serum squamous cell carcinoma antigen in cervical cancer patients based on silver nanoparticles array. *Int J Nanomedicine.* 2014 Feb 22;9:1097–104. Available from: https://pubmed.ncbi.nlm.nih.gov/24591830

19. Monk DJ, Walt DR. Optical fiber-based biosensors. *Anal Bioanal Chem.* 2004 Aug;379(7–8):931–45.

20. Bollella P, Schulz C, Favero G, Mazzei F, Ludwig R, Gorton L, et al. Green synthesis and characterization of gold and silver nanoparticles and their application for development of a third generation lactose biosensor. *Electroanalysis.* 2017;29(1):77–86.

21. Li Y, Schluesener HJ, Xu S. Gold nanoparticle-based biosensors. *Gold Bull.* 2010;43(1):29–41.

22. Antiochia R, Bollella P, Favero G, Mazzei F. Nanotechnology-based surface plasmon resonance affinity biosensors for in vitro diagnostics. *Int J Anal Chem.* 2016;2016:2981931.

23. Choi J-H, Lee J-H, Son J, Choi J-W. Noble metal-assisted surface plasmon resonance immunosensors. *Sensors (Basel).* 2020 Feb 13;20(4):1003. Available from: https://pubmed.ncbi.nlm.nih.gov/32069896

24. Makaraviciute A, Ramanavicius A, Ramanaviciene A. Development of a reusable protein G based SPR immunosensor for direct human growth hormone detection in real samples. *Anal Methods.* 2015;7(23):9875–84. Available from: http://dx.doi.org/10.1039/C5AY01651G

25. Pawula M, Altintas Z, Tothill IE. SPR detection of cardiac troponin T for acute myocardial infarction. *Talanta.* 2016 Jan;146:823–30.

26. Ashaduzzaman M, Deshpande SR, Murugan NA, Mishra YK, Turner APF, Tiwari A. On/off-switchable LSPR nano-immunoassay for troponin-T. *Sci Rep.* 2017 Apr;7:44027.

27. Ben Haddada M, Hu D, Salmain M, Zhang L, Peng C, Wang Y, et al. Gold nanoparticle-based localized surface plasmon immunosensor for staphylococcal enterotoxin A (SEA) detection. *Anal Bioanal Chem.* 2017 Oct;409(26):6227–34.

28. Loiseau A, Zhang L, Hu D, Salmain M, Mazouzi Y, Flack R, et al. Core-shell gold/silver nanoparticles for localized surface plasmon resonance-based naked-eye toxin biosensing. *ACS Appl Mater Interfaces.* 2019 Dec;11(50):46462–71.

29. Lee JU, Nguyen AH, Sim SJ. A nanoplasmonic biosensor for label-free multiplex detection of cancer biomarkers. *Biosens Bioelectron.* 2015 Dec;74:341–6.

30. Aldewachi H, Chalati T, Woodroofe MN, Bricklebank N, Sharrack B, Gardiner P. Gold nanoparticle-based colorimetric biosensors. *Nanoscale.* 2017 Dec;10(1):18–33.

31. Xia N, Deng D, Wang Y, Fang C, Li S-J. Gold nanoparticle-based colorimetric method for the detection of prostate-specific antigen. *Int J Nanomedicine.* 2018;13:2521–30.

32. Shayesteh OH, Ghavami R. A novel label-free colorimetric aptasensor for sensitive determination of PSA biomarker using gold nanoparticles and a cationic polymer in human serum. *Spectrochim Acta A Mol Biomol Spectrosc.* 2020 Feb;226:117644.

33. Lei J, Ju H. Signal amplification using functional nanomaterials for biosensing. *Chem Soc Rev.* 2012 Mar;41(6):2122–34.

34. Brondani D, Piovesan JV, Westphal E, Gallardo H, Fireman Dutra RA, Spinelli A, et al. A label-free electrochemical immunosensor based on an ionic organic molecule and chitosan-stabilized gold nanoparticles for the detection of cardiac troponin T. *Analyst.* 2014 Oct;139(20):5200–8.

35. Rahi A, Sattarahmady N, Heli H. Label-free electrochemical aptasensing of the human prostate-specific antigen using gold nanospears. *Talanta.* 2016 Aug;156–157:218–24.

36. Chinh VD, Speranza G, Migliaresi C, Van Chuc N, Tan VM, Phuong N-T. Synthesis of gold nanoparticles decorated with multiwalled carbon nanotubes (Au-MWCNTs) via cysteaminium chloride functionalization. *Sci Rep.* 2019;9(1):1–9.

37. Heydari-Bafrooei E, Shamszadeh NS. Electrochemical bioassay development for ultrasensitive aptasensing of prostate specific antigen. *Biosens Bioelectron.* 2017 May;91:284–92.

38. Shao H, Lin H, Guo Z, Lu J, Jia Y, Ye M, et al. A multiple signal amplification sandwich-type SERS biosensor for femtomolar detection of miRNA. *Biosens Bioelectron.* 2019 Oct;143:111616.

39. Hamdy ME, Del Carlo M, Hussein HA, Salah TA, El-Deeb AH, Emara MM, et al. Development of gold nanoparticles biosensor for ultrasensitive diagnosis of foot and mouth disease virus. *J Nanobiotechnology.* 2018;16(1):48. Available from: https://doi.org/10.1186/s12951-018-0374-x

40. Hashkavayi AB, Raoof JB. Design an aptasensor based on structure-switching aptamer on dendritic gold nanostructures/Fe(3)O(4)@SiO(2)/DABCO modified screen printed electrode for highly selective detection of epirubicin. *Biosens Bioelectron.* 2017 May;91:650–7.

41. Jin H, Zhao C, Gui R, Gao X, Wang Z. Reduced graphene oxide/nile blue/gold nanoparticles complex-modified glassy carbon electrode used as a sensitive and label-free aptasensor for ratiometric electrochemical sensing of dopamine. *Anal Chim Acta*. 2018 Sep;1025:154–62.

42. Si P, Razmi N, Nur O, Solanki S, Pandey CM, Gupta RK, et al. Gold nanomaterials for optical biosensing and bioimaging. *Nanoscale Adv*. 2021;3(10):2679–98. Available from: http://dx.doi.org/10.1039/D0NA00961J

43. Jain PK, Lee KS, El-Sayed IH, El-Sayed MA. Calculated absorption and scattering properties of gold nanoparticles of different size, shape, and composition: Applications in biological imaging and biomedicine. *J Phys Chem B*. 2006 Apr;110(14):7238–48.

44. Huang X, El-Sayed IH, Qian W, El-Sayed MA. Cancer cell imaging and photothermal therapy in the near-infrared region by using gold nanorods. *J Am Chem Soc*. 2006 Feb;128(6):2115–20.

45. Wan X-Y, Zheng L-L, Gao P-F, Yang X-X, Li C-M, Li YF, et al. Real-time light scattering tracking of gold nanoparticles- bioconjugated respiratory syncytial virus infecting HEp-2 cells. *Sci Rep*. 2014 Mar;4:4529.

46. Sadlowski C, Balderston S, Sandhu M, Hajian R, Liu C, Tran TP, et al. Graphene-based biosensor for on-chip detection of bio-orthogonally labeled proteins to identify the circulating biomarkers of aging during heterochronic parabiosis. *Lab Chip*. 2018 Oct;18(21):3230–8.

47. Wang L, Zhang Y, Wu A, Wei G. Designed graphene-peptide nanocomposites for biosensor applications: A review. *Anal Chim Acta*. 2017 Sep;985:24–40.

48. Ryoo S-R, Yim Y, Kim Y-K, Park I-S, Na H-K, Lee J, et al. High-throughput chemical screening to discover new modulators of microRNA expression in living cells by using graphene-based biosensor. *Sci Rep*. 2018 Jul;8(1):11413.

49. Xie H, Li Y-T, Lei Y-M, Liu Y-L, Xiao M-M, Gao C, et al. Real-time monitoring of nitric oxide at single-cell level with porphyrin-functionalized graphene field-effect transistor biosensor. *Anal Chem*. 2016 Nov;88(22):11115–22.

50. Khalilzadeh B, Shadjou N, Afsharan H, Eskandani M, Nozad Charoudeh H, Rashidi M-R. Reduced graphene oxide decorated with gold nanoparticle as signal amplification element on ultra-sensitive electrochemiluminescence determination of caspase-3 activity and apoptosis using peptide based biosensor. *Bioimpacts*. 2016;6(3):135–47.

51. Tabish TA. Graphene-based materials: The missing piece in nanomedicine? *Biochem Biophys Res Commun*. 2018 Oct;504(4):686–9.

52. Suvarnaphaet P, Pechprasarn S. Graphene-based materials for biosensors: A review. *Sensors*. 2017;17(10):2161.

53. Zeng L, Wang R, Zhu L, Zhang J. Graphene and CdS nanocomposite: A facile interface for construction of DNA-based electrochemical biosensor and its application to the determination of phenformin. *Colloids Surf B Biointerfaces*. 2013 Oct;110:8–14.

54. Li Y, Wang X, Gong J, Xie Y, Wu X, Zhang G. Graphene-based nanocomposites for efficient photocatalytic hydrogen evolution: Insight into the interface toward separation of photogenerated charges. *ACS Appl Mater Interfaces*. 2018 Dec;10(50):43760–7.

55. Li D, Zhang W, Yu X, Wang Z, Su Z, Wei G. When biomolecules meet graphene: From molecular level interactions to material design and applications. *Nanoscale.* 2016 Dec;8(47):19491–509.

56. Liao C, Li Y, Tjong SC. Graphene nanomaterials: Synthesis, biocompatibility, and cytotoxicity. *Int J Mol Sci.* 2018 Nov 12;19(11):3564. Available from: https://pubmed.ncbi.nlm.nih.gov/30424535

57. Korkut S, Roy-Mayhew JD, Dabbs DM, Milius DL, Aksay IA. High surface area tapes produced with functionalized graphene. *ACS Nano.* 2011 Jun;5(6):5214–22.

58. Li H, Wei Q, He J, Li T, Zhao Y, Cai Y, et al. Electrochemical immunosensors for cancer biomarker with signal amplification based on ferrocene functionalized iron oxide nanoparticles. *Biosens Bioelectron.* 2011 Apr;26(8):3590–5.

59. Zhang J, Sun Y, Xu B, Zhang H, Gao Y, Zhang H, et al. A novel surface plasmon resonance biosensor based on graphene oxide decorated with gold nanorod-antibody conjugates for determination of transferrin. *Biosens Bioelectron.* 2013 Jul;45:230–6.

60. Mao K, Wu D, Li Y, Ma H, Ni Z, Yu H, et al. Label-free electrochemical immunosensor based on graphene/methylene blue nanocomposite. *Anal Biochem.* 2012 Mar;422(1):22–7.

61. Wu D, Liu Y, Wang Y, Hu L, Ma H, Wang G, et al. Label-free electrochemiluminescent immunosensor for detection of prostate specific antigen based on aminated graphene quantum dots and carboxyl graphene quantum dots. *Sci Rep.* 2016 Feb;6:20511.

62. Verma S, Singh A, Shukla A, Kaswan J, Arora K, Ramirez-Vick J, et al. Anti-IL8/AuNPs-rGO/ITO as an immunosensing platform for noninvasive electrochemical detection of oral cancer. *ACS Appl Mater Interfaces.* 2017 Aug;9(33):27462–74.

63. Liu F, Gao Y, Li H, Sun S. Interaction of propidium iodide with graphene oxide and its application for live cell staining. *Carbon N Y.* 2014;71:190–5. Available from: https://www.sciencedirect.com/science/article/pii/S0008622314000657

64. Sanginario A, Miccoli B, Demarchi D. Carbon nanotubes as an effective opportunity for cancer diagnosis and treatment. *Biosensors.* 2017;7:9.

65. Chen Y, Zhang Y, Hu Y, Kang L, Zhang S, Xie H, et al. State of the art of single-walled carbon nanotube synthesis on surfaces. *Adv Mater.* 2014 Sep;26(34):5898–922.

66. Noah NM. Design and synthesis of nanostructured materials for sensor applications. *J Nanomater.* 2020;2020:8855321. Available from: https://doi.org/10.1155/2020/8855321

67. Melchionna M, Prato M. Functionalizing carbon nanotubes: An indispensible step towards applications. *ECS J Solid State Sci Technol.* 2013;2(10):M3040–5. Available from: http://dx.doi.org/10.1149/2.008310jss

68. Seeta Rama Raju G, Benton L, Pavitra E, Yu JS. Multifunctional nanoparticles: Recent progress in cancer therapeutics. *Chem Commun.* 2015;51(68):13248–59. Available from: http://dx.doi.org/10.1039/C5CC04643B

69. Thirumalraj B, Kubendhiran S, Chen S-M, Lin K-Y. Highly sensitive electrochemical detection of palmatine using a biocompatible multiwalled carbon nanotube/poly-l-lysine composite. *J Colloid Interface Sci.* 2017;498:144–52. Available from: https://www.sciencedirect.com/science/article/pii/S0021979717302862

70. Lisi S, Scarano S, Fedeli S, Pascale E, Cicchi S, Ravelet C, et al. Toward sensitive immuno-based detection of tau protein by surface plasmon resonance coupled to carbon nanostructures as signal amplifiers. *Biosens Bioelectron.* 2017 Jul;93:289–92.

71. Rezaei B, Shoushtari AM, Rabiee M, Uzun L, Mak WC, Turner APF. An electrochemical immunosensor for cardiac Troponin I using electrospun carboxylated multi-walled carbon nanotube-whiskered nanofibres. *Talanta.* 2018;182:178–86. Available from: https://www.sciencedirect.com/science/article/pii/S0039914018300523

72. Hernández-Rivera M, Zaibaq NG, Wilson LJ. Toward carbon nanotube-based imaging agents for the clinic. *Biomaterials.* 2016 Sep;101:229–40.

73. Sang S, Wang Y, Feng Q, Wei Y, Ji J, Zhang W. Progress of new label-free techniques for biosensors: A review. *Crit Rev Biotechnol.* 2016 May;36(3):465–81.

74. Doucey M-A, Carrara S. Nanowire sensors in cancer. *Trends Biotechnol.* 2019 Jan;37(1):86–99.

75. Cui Y, Wei Q, Park H, Lieber CM. Nanowire nanosensors for highly sensitive and selective detection of biological and chemical species. *Science.* 2001 Aug;293(5533):1289–92.

76. Seker F, Meeker K, Kuech TF, Ellis AB. Surface chemistry of prototypical bulk II–VI and III–V semiconductors and implications for chemical sensing. *Chem Rev.* 2000 Jul;100(7):2505–36.

77. Zhang G-J, Ning Y. Silicon nanowire biosensor and its applications in disease diagnostics: A review. *Anal Chim Acta.* 2012;749:1–15.

78. Tzouvadaki I, Jolly P, Lu X, Ingebrandt S, de Micheli G, Estrela P, et al. Label-free ultrasensitive memristive aptasensor. *Nano Lett.* 2016 Jul;16(7):4472–6.

79. Wang Z, Lee S, Koo K, Kim K. Nanowire-based sensors for biological and medical applications. *IEEE Trans Nanobioscience.* 2016;15(3):186–99.

80. Mu L, Chang Y, Sawtelle SD, Wipf M, Duan X, Reed MA. Silicon nanowire field-effect transistors—A versatile class of potentiometric nanobiosensors. *IEEE Access.* 2015;3:287–302.

81. Li X, Mo J, Fang J, Xu D, Yang C, Zhang M, et al. Vertical nanowire array-based biosensors: Device design strategies and biomedical applications. *J Mater Chem B.* 2020;8(34):7609–32.

82. Liu H, Ruan M, Xiao J, Zhang Z, Chen C, Zhang W, et al. TiO2 nanorod arrays with mesoscopic micro–nano interfaces for in situ regulation of cell morphology and nucleus deformation. *ACS Appl Mater Interfaces.* 2018 Jan;10(1):66–74.

83. Ambhorkar P, Wang Z, Ko H, Lee S, Koo K-I, Kim K, et al. Nanowire-based biosensors: From growth to applications. *Micromachines.* 2018 Dec;9(12):679.

84. Gao Q, Dubrovskii VG, Caroff P, Wong-Leung J, Li L, Guo Y, et al. Simultaneous selective-area and vapor–liquid–solid growth of InP nanowire arrays. *Nano Lett.* 2016 Jul;16(7):4361–7.

85. Hwang YJ, Hahn C, Liu B, Yang P. Photoelectrochemical properties of TiO$_2$ nanowire arrays: A study of the dependence on length and atomic layer deposition coating. *ACS Nano.* 2012 Jun;6(6):5060–9.

86. Kim S, Yoon H, Lee H, Lee S, Jo Y, Lee S, et al. Epitaxy-driven vertical growth of single-crystalline cobalt nanowire arrays by chemical vapor deposition. *J Mater Chem C.* 2015;3(1):100–6.

87. Li C-P, Lee C-S, Ma X-L, Wang N, Zhang R-Q, Lee S-T. Growth direction and cross-sectional study of silicon nanowires. *Adv Mater.* 2003 Apr;15(7–8):607–9.

88. Fan Z, Ho JC, Jacobson ZA, Yerushalmi R, Alley RL, Razavi H, et al. Wafer-scale assembly of highly ordered semiconductor nanowire arrays by contact printing. *Nano Lett.* 2008 Jan;8(1):20–5.

89. Huang Y, Duan X, Wei Q, Lieber CM. Directed assembly of one-dimensional nanostructures into functional networks. *Science.* 2001 Jan;291(5504):630–3.

90. Whang D, Jin S, Wu Y, Lieber CM. Large-scale hierarchical organization of nanowire arrays for integrated nanosystems. *Nano Lett.* 2003 Sep;3(9):1255–9.

91. Yu G, Cao A, Lieber CM. Large-area blown bubble films of aligned nanowires and carbon nanotubes. *Nat Nanotechnol.* 2007;2(6):372–7.

92. Freer EM, Grachev O, Duan X, Martin S, Stumbo DP. High-yield self-limiting single-nanowire assembly with dielectrophoresis. *Nat Nanotechnol.* 2010;5(7):525–30.

93. Huang Z, Geyer N, Werner P, de Boor J, Gösele U. Metal-assisted chemical etching of silicon: A review. *Adv Mater.* 2011 Jan;23(2):285–308.

94. Juhasz R, Elfström N, Linnros J. Controlled fabrication of silicon nanowires by electron beam lithography and electrochemical size reduction. *Nano Lett.* 2005 Feb;5(2):275–80.

95. Mårtensson T, Carlberg P, Borgström M, Montelius L, Seifert W, Samuelson L. Nanowire arrays defined by nanoimprint lithography. *Nano Lett.* 2004 Apr;4(4):699–702.

96. del Campo A, Arzt E. Fabrication approaches for generating complex micro- and nanopatterns on polymeric surfaces. *Chem Rev.* 2008 Mar;108(3):911–45.

97. Wang H, Sun M, Ding K, Hill MT, Ning C-Z. A top-down approach to fabrication of high quality vertical heterostructure nanowire arrays. *Nano Lett.* 2011 Apr;11(4):1646–50.

98. Tian X, Zeng A, Liu Z, Zheng C, Wei Y, Yang P, et al. Carbon quantum dots: In vitro and in vivo studies on biocompatibility and biointeractions for optical imaging. *Int J Nanomedicine.* 2020;15:6519–29.

99. Paul S, Banerjee SL, Khamrai M, Samanta S, Singh S, Kundu PP, et al. Hydrothermal synthesis of gelatin quantum dots for high-performance biological imaging applications. *J Photochem Photobiol B Biol.* 2020;212:112014.

100. Zhang J, Han D, Yang R, Ji Y, Liu J, Yu X. Electrochemical detection of DNA hybridization based on three-dimensional ZnO nanowires/graphite hybrid microfiber structure. *Bioelectrochemistry.* 2019;128:126–32.

101. Pons T, Bouccara S, Loriette V, Lequeux N, Pezet S, Fragola A. In vivo imaging of single tumor cells in fast-flowing bloodstream using near-infrared quantum dots and time-gated imaging. *ACS Nano.* 2019 Mar;13(3):3125–31.

102. Bouccara S, Fragola A, Giovanelli E, Sitbon G, Lequeux N, et al. Time-gated cell imaging using long lifetime near-infrared-emitting quantum dots for autofluorescence rejection. *J Biomed Opt.* 2014;19(5):051208.

103. Zhang Y, Jiang T, Tang L. Near-infrared photoluminescence biosensing platform with gold nanorods-over-gallium arsenide nanohorn array. *Biosens Bioelectron.* 2017;97:278–84.

104. Yasui T, Yanagida T, Shimada T, Otsuka K, Takeuchi M, Nagashima K, et al. Engineering nanowire-mediated cell lysis for microbial cell identification. *ACS Nano.* 2019 Feb;13(2):2262–73.

105. Wu L, Xu X, Sharma B, Wang W, Qu X, Zhu L, et al. Beyond capture: Circulating tumor cell release and single-cell analysis. *Small Methods.* 2019 May;3(5):1800544.

106. Wang S, Wang H, Jiao J, Chen K-J, Owens GE, Kamei K, et al. Three-dimensional nanostructured substrates toward efficient capture of circulating tumor cells. *Angew Chemie Int Ed.* 2009 Nov;48(47):8970–3.

107. Zhang F, Jiang Y, Liu X, Meng J, Zhang P, Liu H, et al. Hierarchical nanowire arrays as three-dimensional fractal nanobiointerfaces for high efficient capture of cancer cells. *Nano Lett.* 2016 Jan;16(1):766–72.

108. Liu X, Chen L, Liu H, Yang G, Zhang P, Han D, et al. Bio-inspired soft polystyrene nanotube substrate for rapid and highly efficient breast cancer-cell capture. *NPG Asia Mater.* 2013;5(9):e63–e63.

109. Feng J, Mo J, Zhang A, Liu D, Zhou L, Hang T, et al. Antibody-free isolation and regulation of adherent cancer cells via hybrid branched microtube-sandwiched hydrodynamic system. *Nanoscale.* 2020;12(8):5103–13.

110. He G, Feng J, Zhang A, Zhou L, Wen R, Wu J, et al. Multifunctional branched nanostraw-electroporation platform for intracellular regulation and monitoring of circulating tumor cells. *Nano Lett.* 2019 Oct;19(10):7201–9.

111. Cai W, Chen X. Nanoplatforms for targeted molecular imaging in living subjects. *Small.* 2007 Nov;3(11):1840–54.

112. Jin S, Hu Y, Gu Z, Liu L, Wu H-C. Application of quantum dots in biological imaging. *J Nanomater.* 2011;2011:834139.

113. Diagaradjane P, Deorukhkar A, Gelovani JG, Maru DM, Krishnan S. Gadolinium chloride augments tumor-specific imaging of targeted quantum dots in vivo. *ACS Nano.* 2010 Jul;4(7):4131–41.

114. Hu J, Wang Z, Li C, Zhang C. Advances in single quantum dot-based nanosensors. Chem Commun. 2017;53(100):13284–95.

115. Wegner KD, Hildebrandt N. Quantum dots: Bright and versatile in vitro and in vivo fluorescence imaging biosensors. *Chem Soc Rev.* 2015;44(14):4792–834.

116. van Sark WGJHM, Frederix PLTM, Van den Heuvel DJ, Gerritsen HC, Bol AA, van Lingen JNJ, et al. Photooxidation and photobleaching of single CdSe/ZnS quantum dots probed by room-temperature time-resolved spectroscopy. *J Phys Chem B.* 2001 Sep;105(35):8281–4.

117. Orte A, Alvarez-Pez JM, Ruedas-Rama MJ. Fluorescence lifetime imaging microscopy for the detection of intracellular ph with quantum dot nanosensors. *ACS Nano.* 2013 Jul;7(7):6387–95.

118. Zamaleeva AI, Collot M, Bahembera E, Tisseyre C, Rostaing P, Yakovlev A V, et al. Cell-penetrating nanobiosensors for pointillistic intracellular Ca^{2+}-transient detection. *Nano Lett.* 2014 Jun;14(6):2994–3001.

119. Ruckh TT, Skipwith CG, Chang W, Senko AW, Bulovic V, Anikeeva PO, et al. Ion-switchable quantum dot förster resonance energy transfer rates in ratiometric potassium sensors. *ACS Nano*. 2016 Apr;10(4):4020–30.

120. Diagaradjane P, Orenstein-Cardona JM, Colón-Casasnovas NE, Deorukhkar A, Shentu S, Kuno N, et al. Imaging epidermal growth factor receptor expression in vivo: Pharmacokinetic and biodistribution characterization of a bioconjugated quantum dot nanoprobe. *Clin Cancer Res*. 2008 Feb;14(3):731–41.

121. Qi L, Gao X. Quantum dot–Amphipol nanocomplex for intracellular delivery and real-time imaging of siRNA. *ACS Nano*. 2008 Jul;2(7):1403–10.

122. Takeda M, Tada H, Higuchi H, Kobayashi Y, Kobayashi M, Sakurai Y, et al. In vivo single molecular imaging and sentinel node navigation by nanotechnology for molecular targeting drug-delivery systems and tailor-made medicine. *Breast Cancer*. 2008;15(2):145–52.

123. Qiao W, Wang B, Wang Y, Yang L, Zhang Y, Shao P. Cancer therapy based on nanomaterials and nanocarrier systems. *J Nanomater*. 2010;2010:796303.

124. Selvan ST. Silica-coated quantum dots and magnetic nanoparticles for bioimaging applications (mini-review). *Biointerphases*. 2010;5(3):FA110–5.

125. Park J-H, Gu L, von Maltzahn G, Ruoslahti E, Bhatia SN, Sailor MJ. Biodegradable luminescent porous silicon nanoparticles for in vivo applications. *Nat Mater*. 2009;8(4):331–6.

126. Gao X, Nie S. Doping mesoporous materials with multicolor quantum dots. *J Phys Chem B*. 2003 Oct;107(42):11575–8.

127. Tilley RD, Yamamoto K. The microemulsion synthesis of hydrophobic and hydrophilic silicon nanocrystals. *Adv Mater*. 2006 Aug;18(15):2053–6.

128. Wang Y, Chang X, Jing N, Zhang Y. Hydrothermal synthesis of carbon quantum dots as fluorescent probes for the sensitive and rapid detection of picric acid. *Anal Methods*. 2018;10(23):2775–84.

129. de Medeiros T V, Manioudakis J, Noun F, Macairan J-R, Victoria F, Naccache R. Microwave-assisted synthesis of carbon dots and their applications. *J Mater Chem C*. 2019;7(24):7175–95.

130. Ang WL, Boon Mee CAL, Sambudi NS, Mohammad AW, Leo CP, Mahmoudi E, et al. Microwave-assisted conversion of palm kernel shell biomass waste to photoluminescent carbon dots. *Sci Rep*. 2020;10(1):21199.

131. Hoang TT, Pham HP, Tran QT. A facile microwave-assisted hydrothermal synthesis of graphene quantum dots for organic solar cell efficiency improvement. *J Nanomater*. 2020;2020:3207909.

132. Architha N, Ragupathi M, Shobana C, Selvankumar T, Kumar P, Lee YS, et al. Microwave-assisted green synthesis of fluorescent carbon quantum dots from Mexican Mint extract for Fe^{3+} detection and bio-imaging applications. *Environ Res*. 2021;199:111263.

133. Hu MZ, Zhu T. Semiconductor nanocrystal quantum dot synthesis approaches towards large-scale industrial production for energy applications. *Nanoscale Res Lett*. 2015 Dec;10(1):469.

134. Ali M, Zayed D, Ramadan W, Kamel OA, Shehab M, Ebrahim S. Synthesis, characterization and cytotoxicity of polyethylene glycol-encapsulated CdTe quantum dots. *Int Nano Lett.* 2019;9(1):61–71.

135. Rajh T, Micic OI, Nozik AJ. Synthesis and characterization of surface-modified colloidal cadmium telluride quantum dots. *J Phys Chem.* 1993 Nov;97(46):11999–2003.

136. Ndangili PM, Jijana AM, Baker PGL, Iwuoha EI. 3-Mercaptopropionic acid capped ZnSe quantum dot-cytochrome P450 3A4 enzyme biotransducer for 17β-estradiol. *J Electroanal Chem.* 2011;653(1–2):67–74.

137. Masikini M, Ndangili PM, Ikpo CO, Feleni U, Duoman S, Sidwaba U, et al. Optoelectronics of stochiometrically controlled palladium telluride quantum dots. *J Nano Res.* 2016;40:29–45.

138. Ndangili PM, Olowu RA, Mailu SN, Ngece RF, Jijana A, Williams A, et al. Impedimetric response of a label-free genosensor prepared on a 3-mercaptopropionic acid capped gallium selenide nanocrystal modified gold electrode. *Int J Electrochem Sci.* 2011;6(5):1438–53.

139. Ndangili PM, Masikini M, Feleni U, Douman S, Tovide O, Williams A, et al. Gallium-induced perturbation of zinc selenide quantum dots electronics. *ChemistrySelect.* 2017;2(24):7054–62.

140. Ndangili PM, Arotiba OA, Baker PGL, Iwuoha EI. A potential masking approach in the detection of dopamine on 3-mercaptopropionic acid capped ZnSc quantum dots modified gold electrode in the presence of interferences. *J Electroanal Chem.* 2010;643(1–2):77–81.

141. Afsari HS, Cardoso Dos Santos M, Lindén S, Chen T, Qiu X, van Bergen en Henegouwen PMP, et al. Time-gated FRET nanoassemblies for rapid and sensitive intra- and extracellular fluorescence imaging. *Sci Adv.* 2016 Jun;2(6):e1600265.

142. Mandal G, Darragh M, Wang YA, Heyes CD. Cadmium-free quantum dots as time-gated bioimaging probes in highly-autofluorescent human breast cancer cells. *Chem Commun.* 2013;49(6):624–6.

143. Molaei MJ. Carbon quantum dots and their biomedical and therapeutic applications: A review. *RSC Adv.* 2019;9(12):6460–81.

144. Whitlow J, Pacelli S, Paul A. Multifunctional nanodiamonds in regenerative medicine: Recent advances and future directions. *J Control Release.* 2017;261:62–86.

145. Jaiswal JK, Mattoussi H, Mauro JM, Simon SM. Long-term multiple color imaging of live cells using quantum dot bioconjugates. *Nat Biotechnol.* 2003;21(1):47–51.

146. Li H, Shih WY, Shih W-H. Synthesis and characterization of aqueous carboxyl-capped CdS quantum dots for bioapplications. *Ind Eng Chem Res.* 2007 Mar;46(7):2013–9.

147. Hyun B-R, Chen, Rey DA, Wise FW, Batt CA. Near-infrared fluorescence imaging with water-soluble lead salt quantum dots. *J Phys Chem B.* 2007 May;111(20):5726–30.

148. Duan H, Nie S. Cell-penetrating quantum dots based on multivalent and endosome-disrupting surface coatings. *J Am Chem Soc.* 2007 Mar;129(11):3333–8.

Index